OVERSATURATED

OVERSATURATED

A GUIDE TO CONVERSATIONS ABOUT FATS WITH YOUR PATIENTS

EVAN ALLEN, MD

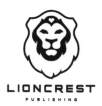

LIONCREST
PUBLISHING

OVERSATURATED
A Guide to Conversations about Fats with Your Patients

ISBN   978-1-5445-0336-3 *Paperback*
       978-1-5445-0337-0 *Ebook*

I dedicate this book to my son, Ryndon, with hopes he will grow up in a world with substantially fewer needless deaths.

CONTENTS

ACKNOWLEDGMENTS

The information and messages in this book are based on the work and guidance I've received from the doctors and scientists who have taken the time to read the clinical literature and help me interpret it. This includes Dr. John McDougall, Dr. Dean Ornish, Dr. Caldwell Esselstyn, Raymond J. Cronise, Dr. Michael Greger, Dr. Joel Fuhrman, Dr. Garth Davis, Evelyn Kocur from the Carbsane blog, Plant Positive from his YouTube Channel, Seth Yoder, and many others who have studied the scientific literature and see the benefits of a plant-based diet low in saturated fat.

INTRODUCTION

TALK ABOUT A BAD DIET

I recently attended a medical lecture where a rheumatol-ogist was discussing how he treats gout.

Gout is an excruciating form of arthritis caused when razor-sharp uric acid crystals form in the joints. Patients with gout often put their pain level at a nine or ten on a scale of ten. Their joints feel like they are caught in a tightening vise and become red, swollen, and exqui-sitely tender.

Gout can lead to permanent joint damage and deformi-ties. Worse, the condition is associated with much higher risks of renal failure, diabetes, and cancer. People with gout are also more likely to have heart disease, high blood pressure, blocked arteries, and heart failure. Avoiding gout in the first place is way better than getting a single attack.

Gout hits most often when people consume a lot of shellfish, red meat, lamb, pork, beer, or other grain liquors. Saturated fats, including those found in cheese, butter, dairy products, and red meat, reduce the body's ability to eliminate the uric acid that crystallizes in the joints.

So, if you're a doctor treating a patient with gout, you're likely to have a conversation with your patient about diet, right?

I mean, wouldn't you?

Maybe.

Maybe not.

At the lecture I attended, the rheumatologist told us that as long as we put our gout patients on the right medicine, we don't even need to bother advising them on diet.

Wait...what?

You're saying we shouldn't talk to a patient about food

when their diet is giving them level-nine pain and putting them at risk of life-threatening metabolic disease?

MAKING THINGS LESS BAD

I can't say I was surprised to hear the rheumatologist say this. Most of us treating patients today steer away from advising them on diet and nutrition, even when that nutritional advice is completely uncontroversial and scientifically proven to help them.

Instead, we're content to treat patients' symptoms with drugs or surgery. Rather than reducing the incidence of disease, the healthcare professions have quietly accepted the goal of merely making things less bad. We can slow down the pace of metabolic illnesses like heart disease or diabetes, but we've given up trying to prevent, halt, or reverse them.

Dr. Denis Burkitt once asked colleagues to imagine a crowd of people running toward a cliff; if they run past the edge and fall, they are horribly injured or killed. As healthcare practitioners, much of what we are doing seems like stacking pillow top mattresses at the bottom to soften the landing. Some patients survive, but they've still fallen off the cliff and are left to deal with the aftermath of their injuries.[1]

I often tell patients that the best heart attack is the one you don't get. The least damaging stroke is about a thousand times worse than not having a stroke. The least dangerous case of prostate cancer is the one you never get.

Yet how many of us in the healthcare profession spend the bulk of our time reducing the likelihood of these diseases? Yes, we give statins and treat blood pressure, but often by the point we do that, significant damage has already occurred.

The role of healthcare should be to prevent people from even approaching that cliff. At the very least, medical professionals should aim to erect a fence at the top to help prevent people from falling.

To me, the fence represents behavior: diet, exercise, and avoiding known poisons. For that fence to be effective, we need to sink some sturdy posts. A patient shouldn't smoke, for instance. That's one post. Patients shouldn't drink alcohol in excess either. That's another post.

Another critical fencepost is diet. We are not building a sturdy fence if we don't address food and specifically deal with the overconsumption of saturated fat. Alcohol and smoking are simply metabolically harmful substances that we put in our bodies.

Saturated fat, contrary to a narrative that has emerged over the last decade, falls into the same category.

THE TRUTH ABOUT SATURATED FAT

Saturated fats increase the dangerous cholesterol (LDL) and the Apo(b)[2] in your bloodstream and cause blockages in your arteries, leading to heart attacks and strokes.[3] Plaque forms on the interior walls of your arteries, causing blood flow to decrease, while pressure in the vessel goes up.

This artery-shrinking occurs through the whole body. The blood flow to the tiny bones in your ears is reduced, diminishing your hearing[4]. For men, blood flow to your penis gets sluggish, causing erectile dysfunction[5]—something that affects about 40 percent of the men over fifty in our country today.[6] Low blood flow to connective tissues leads to injuries, such as torn Achilles tendons and rotator cuffs.[7] People who eat a lot of saturated fat have a greater incidence of lower back pain[8], diabetes[9], and dementia.[10]

A diet rich in saturated fat, which is found in baked goods, pizza, beef, pork, lamb, salami, sausages, chicken skin, tropical oils, fried foods, and such dairy products as regular-fat milk, cheese, cream, and butter, can also make you obese[11]. And obesity comes with its own host of metabolic problems, including diabetes, heart disease, stroke, some cancers, gallbladder disease, gallstones, osteoarthritis, sleep apnea, and, of course, gout.[12]

It's not a secret.

The US Department of Agriculture's dietary guidelines say we should limit saturated fat to less than 10 percent of our daily caloric intake. The American Heart Association recommends keeping it to 6 percent or less. Unfortunately, saturated fat is so prevalent in the American diet that it is almost impossible to avoid. Even nondairy creamer has saturated fat in it. Anyone who wants to limit saturated fat has to be extraordinarily vigilant.

However, it is worth the effort. Study after study[13] in the last several decades shows that strictly limiting saturated fat reduces the risk of heart and vascular problems. When they reduce their consumption of saturated fat, even healthy, fit, and trim individuals get as much benefit as patients with high blood pressure, high cholesterol, or diabetes. The greater the reduction in saturated fat, the greater the protection from heart and vascular problems.

Reducing intake of saturated fat doesn't merely prevent these health problems and save lives; it can reverse existing health problems. In my medical practice, in addition to losing weight and feeling more energetic, we get patients off Viagra and insulin when they improve their diet and reduce their saturated fat.

WHY THE MESSAGE ISN'T GETTING THROUGH

Despite a mountain of scientific evidence that we should

restrict saturated fat in our diets, the message isn't reaching our patients. One reason is that many doctors are confused about what to say on the subject. They remember what they learned in school—that a diet high in saturated fats leads to obesity, heart disease, and a wide variety of metabolic problems—but in recent years, partly due to a campaign waged by the food industry and its allies, they've heard conflicting information and now don't feel confident talking about it.

It's no surprise that the message about saturated fat has become muddled in recent years. Trade groups whose products are rich in saturated fat have worked hard to distort the truth by funding research to support their products.

A recent research paper that said a diet rich in eggs did no more harm to a person's vascular system than a diet rich in oatmeal was funded by the Egg Nutrition Center, whose motto is "Credible Science, Incredible Egg" and whose primary funder is the American Egg Board.[14] A recent study on the beneficial effects of a high-fat meat and high-fat cheese diet on HDL was funded by the Dairy Research Institute and the Danish Dairy Research Foundation.[15]

These studies—and there are dozens of them—are designed to narrowly focus on the benefits of these products and not the risks associated with them. While these studies are often conducted by reputable researchers—David Katz of Yale's Yale-Griffin Prevention Research Center has done research for the ENC—other studies have shown that more than 90 percent of nutritional studies conducted with food industry funding come out with a finding that favors the funders.[16]

If a study funded by R.J. Reynolds concluded that secondhand cigarette smoke was healthy, would you believe it? If Exxon funds a study on global warming, would you trust the result?

Of course you wouldn't.

So why would you believe studies on diet funded by the Cattleman's Beef Association? Or the National Dairy Council?

Another reason for this confusion is the way media handle the propaganda generated by these conflict-laden reports. The media tend to amplify messages that don't rock the boat ("A new study says that cheese omelet you love poses no more danger to your arteries than a bowl of granola!") and minimize messages that suggest your habits are killing you. Why would a TV station that runs millions of dollars in advertising for Arby's ("We have the meats!") look hard at a study suggesting you limit your fast-food meals to annual splurges?

The goal of these tainted food-industry studies isn't to directly suggest that saturated fat is beneficial but instead to sow doubt and confusion. (Great! Eggs are OK to eat now!)

Since most people classify foods as "good" or "bad," when researchers declare something "not bad," most consumers will perceive those foods as "good."

People gladly accept any reason to continue doing what they enjoy. They don't like to make big behavioral changes. It takes a strong case made in a compelling way for you to change your behavior.

That is my purpose for this book.

GETTING TO THE TRUTH

I'm writing this book to give healthcare professionals the clear, unvarnished truth about saturated fat. They can then communicate it to their patients with confidence and the right amount of urgency. I pored over a century worth of research so you don't have to, and the more I examined how the science and media messages ("Butter may, in fact, be back," *Time* magazine crowed in 2016) camouflaged the danger of saturated fat, the more convinced I became that this book was needed.

When I went to Amazon to search for a book that explained the dangers of eating saturated fat, I couldn't find one. In fact, the first twenty books all advocated diets rich in fat and took the position that dietary guidelines about saturated fat are all bunk! It was like searching for books about geography and finding twenty books by planaterrists (people who believe the Earth is flat).

I also realized that if those of us in healthcare are to develop a consistent message about the dangers of saturated fat, we must adopt these changes ourselves. Back in the fifties, tobacco companies used doctors to advertise their products, and many doctors had ashtrays in their exam rooms. But today less than 2 percent of doctors smoke. The most significant social change that came about with smoking in the general public is a result not of doctors advising their patients to stop smoking, but of doctors themselves not smoking.

I want the same kind of change for saturated fat. As healers, our disdain for saturated fat needs to be nearly as pervasive and persistent as our contempt for cigarette smoking.

FAKE NEWS ABOUT FATS

From 1994 to about 2010, I was seeing up to sixty patients a day. Most doctors see ten to fifteen, but I worked on military bases and hospitals, and at nights I moonlighted at urgent care facilities. I treated hospital patients, delivered babies, and scrubbed in for more surgeries than I care to count. I helped thousands of people, but the work was often unsatisfying to me.

That's because I felt like I wasn't making a lasting difference in my patients' lives. When you work in an emergency room and a patient comes in with a heart attack and you successfully break up the blood clot, you save someone's life. That's great! You're a hero! But you've done nothing to stop them from coming back in six months with the same problem. That bothered me.

Then, when I was in my mid-forties, I became ill myself. I was a lifelong vegetarian, but I was also obese. I was diagnosed with nonalcoholic steatohepatitis, or fatty liver, which is the gateway to cirrhosis and liver failure. I had recurring urticarial vasculitis, asthma, and sleep apnea. I wheezed regularly and had elevated liver enzymes and cholesterol. I couldn't get the life insurance policy I wanted because of my health. At the time I thought, "Wait a minute. How can this be? I do everything I advise my patients to do; why am I getting metabolic disease?"

A friend suggested I watch *Forks Over Knives*, a documentary film about the work of Drs. T. Colin Campbell, PhD; John McDougall, MD; Dean Ornish, MD; and Caldwell

Esselstyn, MD, and others whose research concluded that heart disease, type 2 diabetes, and several forms of cancer could be prevented or reversed through a whole-food, plant-based diet. Based on their research all over the world, these researchers and practicing doctors recommended a diet of whole, unrefined plants including fruits, vegetables, tubers, whole grains, and legumes. The diet minimized meat, including chicken and fish, dairy products, eggs, oil, and refined flour and sugar.

The film was particularly critical of oils. They felt all oils damage blood vessels and promote bleeding by thinning the blood. In addition to adding loads of calories, oils also hurt lung function and oxygen exchange, suppressed certain immune system functions, and increased cancer risk.

The core message of the film is that much of what is going on in medicine today is fixable by changing nutritional patterns. This ran counter to the commonly accepted belief, still prevalent today, that many metabolic diseases are genetic, which means there isn't much you can do; if your mom and dad had diabetes, you're probably going to get it, too.

I was skeptical about the film.

I had read all the same headlines about nutrition and fats you have. I knew people who swore by their high-fat, ketogenic diets and drank bulletproof coffee (rich in butter, but only from grass-fed cows). I doubted that the film had taken into account all this new evidence coming out about how great eggs and olive oil are for you, which I was eating regularly to add animal protein to my vegetarian diet.

But then I started researching the details. I read books and pored over journal articles. I started analyzing these so-called "new findings" about fat, and when I did, I realized that most of the recent research was propaganda.

Fake news.

It wasn't real science at all. Instead, industry money was being used to shape a consensus, and people like me had swallowed it.

The reality was the evidence supporting a low-saturated-fat diet was overpowering and substantial. It went back a century and was utterly convincing. These new studies were not challenging those findings but instead were using statistical methods that we could predict in advance would show the results they obtained, using the methods developed over the last century. This led them to half-baked results that cast doubt on the more reputable science. These pseudo-studies were seemingly designed to result in misleading headlines ("Breakfast gourmands who fear ill effects of eggs can cast off their yolks of burden") and TV interviews with nonmedical "health experts" espousing the value of coconut oil. These advocates were often funded by food industry trade groups.

As a result of my research, I cut saturated fats, eggs, and dairy from my vegetarian diet and focused on high-fiber foods. Within six months, I'd lost forty-five pounds, and my asthma and urticarial vasculitis went away. Within a year, I was able to get a new insurance policy and saved a considerable amount of money as a result.

I began to advise my patients differently. Some people followed my advice, and some followed it a little bit. Over time, I found that the results my patients saw correlated with the amount of effort they put into changing their eating habits. Those who did the most reliably got the best results.

AN HONEST ASSESSMENT

This book is not a diet book. I'm not trying to convince you to follow a specific prescribed eating program, either. There are no recipes for banana bread, and I'm not coming out with a companion cookbook. It's not a personal memoir of my health struggles or how I conquered them when I changed my diet.

Instead, it's an honest overview of the risks associated

with a diet high in saturated fat. We'll take a hard look at both the underlying science and the faux science that's been used to undercut the dangers of saturated fats and cloud the risks. As I dug into these issues and reviewed decades of scientific research, I looked for a straightforward resource that explained these issues in plain language, but I couldn't find one.

We need one.

The conversation in social, print, and television media today is dominated by industry propaganda, but if those of us in the medical field have a resource that sorts the science from the disinformation, we will be more likely to change our own behaviors while convincing our patients to do the same.

This book will examine the following issues:

- **Chapter 1: A Mountain of Evidence.** Researchers have developed ironclad evidence about the dangers of diets high in saturated fat.
- **Chapter 2: Trouble with Change.** How food industry spin doctors have manipulated science to convince people to continue buying milk, cheese, red meat, and other products rich in this deadly saturated fat.
- **Chapter 3: A Dangerous Meal.** The true scope of

the public health dilemma posed by diets full of saturated fat.

- **Chapter 4: Managing Cholesterol.** Why LDL cholesterol is still a pervasive danger in the US and how diets rich in saturated fats make it worse.
- **Chapter 5: Diabetes: Simple Answers for Complex Chemistry.** The best way to fight diabetes is to reduce your intake of saturated fats.
- **Chapter 6: Ceramides.** Like cholesterol, these big, sticky molecules produced from saturated fat play a role in diabetes, heart disease, and cancer.
- **Chapter 7: Dementia.** Saturated fat decreases blood flow to both the heart *and* the brain. The results can be devastating.
- **Chapter 8: When Communities Change How They Eat.** We'll go from Finland and Denmark to Cuba and Southeast Asia to see the benefits of a diet that is very low in saturated fat.
- **Chapter 9: Talking to Your Patients.** How to help your patients find the right balance.

WHERE WE'RE HEADED

This book will help you do your job—get people healthy. It will help you cut through the half-truths about saturated fat and give you the confidence to deliver honest, down-to-earth, and indisputable advice to your patients. If patients keep hearing the same things over and over from healthcare professionals, it's going to be increasingly difficult for them to believe the internet guru or diet book advising them to get 40 percent of their calories from saturated fat.

Along the way, I also hope to convince you to change some of your own habits.

If you're like me and feel like you are just helping patients feel less bad, I hope this book gives you some optimism. We can do this. I've seen it happen.

Together, we can put up warning signs and build a sturdy fence that prevents patients from running off that cliff. Are you ready to start?

Chapter 1

A MOUNTAIN OF EVIDENCE AGAINST SATURATED FAT

The first medical description of vascular disease was recorded in the late 1700s. At the time, the disease was rare and would remain that way for decades. Doctors in the 1800s who discovered patients with atherosclerosis would get excited because the problem was uncommon and the cause was a mystery. These doctors noticed that the disease—in which plaque forms in arteries and constricts the flow of blood—primarily showed up in wealthy people with rich diets. Poor people, who at the time survived on spartan diets and had average body mass indexes of 18 to 19—shockingly thin by modern standards—simply did not get vascular disease.

Heart disease and stroke didn't become a more widespread problem until the late 1800s when our food system began to be industrialized. Before refrigeration and other modern conveniences, most Americans' diets were based on the food they purchased in burlap sacks from dry good stores—grains and flour—which they mixed with vegetables and fruit they got at farmers' markets. Large amounts of fresh meat and dairy were out of the price range of most. People couldn't consume large amounts of saturated fat because they didn't have easy access to it, and even if they did, they couldn't afford it.

Modern factories, refrigeration, and electricity changed that. With technology, people could store a greater variety of food—including meat, dairy products, and eggs—over a longer period. Those foods typically have higher caloric and fat content, and as these foods became a bigger part of our diet, vascular disease became much more common.

We see the same pattern in every country that becomes industrialized, regardless of when that happens: death rates initially plummet because people get fewer infectious diseases and hygiene and medical treatment improve. Infant mortality drops dramatically. People put on weight. They get fat and happy, for the most part.

But then, about a decade or so after the food system changes, older people start showing signs of heart disease and diabetes. Because these diseases come on gradually, health and medical officials often don't connect the problem to long-term changes in their patients' diet. However, looking back, you can see the relationship between dietary changes and widespread increases in noncommunicable diseases.

One of the best examples we have is the experience of the Irish in the late 1800s. After the potato famine, people stopped eating oatmeal and potatoes and started consuming store-bought jams, biscuits, and bacon. The percentage of their calories from fat rose from less than 5 percent of their diet—and in many cases much lower—to 27 percent. Cases of diabetes and vascular diseases skyrocketed as the Irish intake of saturated fat increased.[17]

If drastically cutting our consumption of carbohydrates and increasing our intake of fat were ideal—as books like Gary Taubes's *Good Calories, Bad Calories* recommend—then we should have seen an epidemic of chronic diseases in the 1800s, when everybody ate a high carbohydrate diet. Imagine Oliver Twist and his fellow orphans getting chubby on their gruel. This is the world that we should see if Taubes's book were correct.

Instead, history shows the opposite. The rate of diabetes climbed nearly 6,000 percent in Ireland when fat consumption increased, replacing potatoes in the average diet.[18]

China is another excellent example. The Chinese had a largely agrarian, nonindustrial economy until about 1980. As it became industrialized, the rate of diabetes and obesity increased. Today, China's rate of diabetes is higher than the US rate, and its obesity rates are starting to track closely with other industrialized nations. More Chinese are dying from vascular disease than ever before.[19] Since the development of China's industrial food system, the percentage of carbohydrates in the typical Chinese diet has declined from 80 percent to 55 percent and the percentage of calories from fat has tripled.[20] KFC, McDonald's, and Starbucks have opened thousands of new outlets and continue to expand.[21] A study in the scientific journal *Nutrients* found that China has shifted away from its traditional diet to a high-fat, low-carbohydrate, and low-fiber diet with fewer nutrients than the American diet. As carbohydrate consumption went down and fat consumption went up, the percentage of the population that is overweight went from 11 percent in 1991 to nearly 30 percent in 2009.[22]

Researchers have a name for when a developing country moves from a traditional diet high in cereal and fiber to more Western diets rich in sugars, fat, and animal-source food. It's called the nutritional transition. Countries aren't as afflicted with high rates of infectious disease, starvation, and malnutrition as before, but within fifteen years are experiencing previously unknown levels of metabolic disorders associated with the rich new diets.

With the economic development of China and India, the bulk of the world's population has nearly completed the transition to an industrialized food system, and as a result, the number-one cause of death on the planet is heart disease and it has been for decades.[23]

FINDING THE FAT LINK

By the early 1900s, nations like the United States that had adopted an industrialized food system experienced an epidemic of vascular disease. Lots of people started dropping dead from heart attacks and strokes, which until that point were much more rare.

Trying to examine the problem, scientists and physicians fed diets high in saturated fat and/or cholesterol to mammals and saw that the animals developed the same arterial changes that humans on similar diets exhibited. Plaque clogged the animals' arteries, and the plaque building up in the animals' arteries was identical to the plaque researchers found in people with vascular disease.

In 1913, Nikolai N. Anitschkov, a physician in the Russian army, became the first researcher to find the link between atherosclerosis and dietary cholesterol. He fed one group of rabbits purified cholesterol in sunflower oil and a second group just sunflower oil. After three or four months, he observed in the cholesterol-treated rabbits the same vascular lesions you find in humans with atherosclerosis. The rabbits not given cholesterol showed no lesions. Anitschkov got the same results with guinea pigs.

Researchers later found that diets high in saturated fats but lacking cholesterol also created plaque in arteries. If your food has a lot of cholesterol, it raises your low-density lipoprotein (LDL—the dangerous cholesterol). But saturated fat makes your liver create lots more cholesterol, raising LDL levels.[24]

You have limited resources for getting rid of LDL. The body can only eliminate about 500 milligrams a day in feces. That's a tiny amount—something on the order of one-thousandth of a teaspoon. Since most people eat more than that, the body squirrels it away in different places. One place is the walls of your arteries, but there are other places too. People with genetically high cholesterol can get odd tumors on their skin or white patches in the middle parts of their eyes. These are other pockets of stored cholesterol.

The work of Anitschkov and others has been replicated

thousands of times in the hundred years since these early discoveries. Twenty-five different species of mammals have been fed diets high in saturated fat and all got vascular disease. Not once have omnivorous animals fed a high saturated fat diet emerged from the study with low levels of cholesterol and low rates of vascular disease. It doesn't matter whether the saturated fat comes from butter or lard or from plant-based sources such as tropical oils. The purified coconut oil that many researchers use as a source of saturated fat behaves just as bad or worse than lard, butter, or trans fat in producing atherosclerosis.

It's not the food source.

It's the saturated fat.

THE HEART DISEASE EPIDEMIC

By the later 1940s and early 1950s, heart disease in the United States was an epidemic. Politicians keeled over in Congress giving speeches. As Taubes relates in *Good Calories, Bad Calories*, President Dwight Eisenhower dropped on the golf course one day with a heart attack. Taubes doesn't mention that Eisenhower ate sausages, bacon, and hotcakes for breakfast that morning and a hamburger with raw onions for lunch. Ulcer patients put on a diet of heavy cream, eggs, farina, and butter called the Sippey diet had twice as many heart attacks as other ulcer patients not given the diet.[25]

There was no mystery about what was happening, or what was causing it. Scientists had closed in on the effects of dietary cholesterol and saturated fat so precisely that they could accurately predict the increase in a patient's cholesterol reading based on what the patient ate using equations verified in research around the world. Researchers had done thousands of animal studies, hundreds of epidemiological studies, and several hundred metabolic ward studies, and all the pieces of the puzzle fit together. In addition, when observations were made of people, those restricting saturated fat had lower heart attack rates.

Unfortunately, the word wasn't getting out to consumers.

Part of the problem was the United State Department of Agriculture's dietary guidelines at the time. Many of you (including me) may be too young to remember, but in 1956 the USDA released a food guide[26] that recommended that we eat from four food groups—milk, meat, grain products, and fruit and vegetables. The "Basic Four" guide remained in effect for more than twenty years, and the USDA didn't really highlight the role saturated fat played in chronic disease until 1979, several decades after the research on this topic was crystal-clear.

Why did it take so long? If doctors and scientists knew that saturated fat from tropical oils, eggs, meat, fish, and dairy caused health problems, why was the government recommending we eat it?

The answer is pretty obvious.

It was necessary to sell the goods being produced by American farmers. Promoting the sale of agricultural products has always been the USDA's primary job, and they did it without apology. The conflict came when we asked the same agency that promotes sales to also set our dietary guidelines. The USDA couldn't promote beef one minute and discourage its consumption the next, so it has focused on increasing consumption of food products like milk, cheese, and meat.

To this day, the USDA runs a program called commodity checkoff, where it collects taxes from the sales of commodities and uses them to do things like get fast food restaurants to add more cheese to their menus or run ads on your TV calling pork "The Other White Meat." The only significant agricultural commodity that doesn't have a program is chicken, but since consumption of chicken has gone up 600 percent over the last century,[27] the USDA help hasn't been needed.[28]

Another factor was what we considered normal levels of

cholesterol. In the 1950s, you were considered to have high cholesterol if your cholesterol was over 300 milligrams per deciliter. That's staggeringly high. Today, either 200 or 240 mg/dl is viewed as the cutoff, and total cholesterol levels less than 200 are deemed to be okay for adults. Even that number is too high, however. The normal cholesterol for human populations not afflicted with a heart disease epidemic (typically those groups that haven't made the nutrition transition) is 150 or lower, and a normal LDL cholesterol in those populations is between 50 and 70.

Although today's recommended cholesterol levels remain too high, the drop in the recommended levels in the 1960s helped stem the epidemic of heart disease. Doctors and patients took steps to lower those cholesterol readings, and in the 1980s, statin drugs and improved techniques for heart disease care also reduced the number of deaths.

The average cholesterol levels for the country declined. One study that looked at the autopsies of young male soldiers killed in the Korean, Vietnam, and Afghanistan wars showed the evidence of coronary atherosclerosis declined from 77 percent of the soldiers serving in Korea (1950-53), to 45 percent of the American casualties in Vietnam (1968-78) to 8.5 percent in the Middle East in the 2000s, an undeniably massive improvement.[29]

But the improvements in cholesterol levels came too late for some. Eisenhower's heart attack struck on the eighth hole of a golf course outside Denver in 1955 when the former Supreme Allied Commander in Europe was in his first term as president. Eisenhower loved eating meat, and he also loved cigarettes, and he didn't religiously follow the restrictive diet his doctors put him on. He ate a lot of Emdee, which was a processed fat product made from artery-clogging hydrogenated coconut oil[30] that was marketed by the pharmaceutical company Pitman-Moore. Eisenhower also continued to smoke after his heart attack and suffered a stroke a year after his re-election in 1956. All told, he suffered seven myocardial infarctions and fourteen cardiac arrests before he died in 1969 at the age of seventy-eight.

WHEN COMMUNITIES CHANGED

The correlation between saturated fat and cardiovascular disease was solidified in the 1950s when Ancel Keys, a University of California, Berkeley and Harvard-trained physiologist working at the University of Minnesota, noticed a counterintuitive fact: wealthy and well-fed American business executives had high rates of heart disease while impoverished residents of post-war Europe had sharply declining rates of heart disease. The countries with the least amount of average dietary fat had the lowest rates of heart disease.

Keys was already a widely known researcher (he designed K-rations used in World War II). To test his hypothesis, he created a longitudinal cohort study that came to be known as the Seven Countries Study (SCS). The study, which is ongoing, had found by 1970 that a Mediterranean-style diet low in animal fat protected against heart disease.[31]

When first published, the SCS found that Finland had the highest level of saturated fat consumption in the studied cohorts and that Japan had the lowest. Not surprisingly, the heart disease rate in Finland was twenty times greater than Japan's. The Finns weren't happy with these findings, but rather than attack the science, they attacked the problem by launching a "Dairy to Berries" project in the 1970s shortly after the SCS was published that encouraged residents to replace butter, dairy, and meat in their diets with unprocessed plant food, such as the berries that grow abundantly in the region.

The result?

In the North Karelia region of Finland where the project started, researchers recorded a 73 percent reduction in heart disease deaths. It was an astounding number.

And it didn't go unnoticed.

The United States Senate Select Committee on Nutrition

and Human Needs, headed by Senator George McGovern, reviewed data from the Seven Countries Study, the research already done on the dangers of cholesterol and saturated fat, and the epidemiological and demographic studies conducted around the globe. In January 1977, the committee issued a new set of nutritional guidelines that recommended that Americans eat less processed sugar, high-fat meat, egg, and dairy products and more "complex carbohydrates," such as fruits, vegetables, and whole grains as a way to prevent the "diseases of civilization" such as heart disease, stroke, certain cancers, high blood pressure, obesity, diabetes, and generalized atherosclerosis.

Not surprisingly, this triggered a backlash from the meat, dairy, egg, and sugar industries, and the committee's revised final recommendations were severely watered down. Mention of specific foods was shelved in favor of recommendations to reduce "saturated fat" which at that time few people even understood. McGovern blamed these special interests for derailing his re-election campaign in South Dakota.

The committee's work led to new dietary guidelines from the United States Center for Nutrition Policy and Promotion. Yet to this day, this agency of the USDA continues to be accused of favoring the food industry over the public's interest in clear, science-based dietary advice.

The result is that Americans and even some of their healthcare providers remain largely confused about saturated fat and where it comes from. Some think that most of their dietary saturated fat comes from meat, but in truth, most of the saturated fat in the American diet comes from cheese, pizza, baked goods, and dairy products, not meat.[32] That means many vegetarians, like I was, think they've reduced their intake of saturated fat because they eschew meat—an erroneous assumption since saturated fat comes from a wide variety of foods, including the tropical oils used heavily in many vegetarian and vegan products.

THE CASE IS IRREFUTABLE

The evidence regarding the health risks from eating too much saturated fat is mountainous. It's not necessarily new information—although in future chapters we'll discuss recent findings that raise new concerns—but the dangers from saturated fat have been backed up time and again through every type of double-blind, clinical, epidemiological, and metabolic ward study you can imagine. Even an 800-page tome would fail to document it all, and sadly, few would read it.

The case against saturated fat is so irrefutable that it's akin to Newton's Laws of Motion. Einstein came along and developed a more complex understanding of relativity, but Newton's laws remain solid science. You can conduct all of Newton's experiments today and they all still work. Later research merely allowed us to understand more deeply why they work.

The same is true for our knowledge about saturated fat. We have known for decades that diets high in saturated fat are closely linked with the development of all these horrible illnesses, and in the last ten to twenty years, even more evidence has explained the mechanisms through which saturated fat harms the body.

The benefits of strictly limiting your consumption of saturated fat are so far-reaching that it seems almost too good to be true. If a stockbroker promised you a 30 percent return on your investment, you'd think the offer was a scam. But the benefit to people of limiting saturated fat dwarfs that 30 percent return and has been medically proven to work. For patients at risk of noncommunicable metabolic disorders, including heart attacks, strokes, diabetes, hypertension, and fatty liver, the first order of business for a medical practitioner is to talk to those patients about their diet, especially the saturated fat in that diet.

When I talk to patients, their eyes light up when I describe the nutrition transition we see in the world. Most of them understand that when more processed, higher-fat foods become available, people get sicker.

When countries shift to an industrialized food system, their saturated fat consumption climbs, and the metabolic problems appear like clockwork. It never fails. Good science makes predictions that are borne out when tested. It's the most irrefutable evidence there is. And when populations purposely lower their saturated fat consumption—as the population of Finland did (see chapter 8 for more details)—deaths from metabolic problems plummet dramatically.

If saturated fat consumption were an unalloyed benefit—as many nonscientific modern books suggest—we would see the exact opposite. The people of Finland would never have bothered with its Dairy to Berries project because they wouldn't have needed it, they would have been the healthiest cohort in SCS.

The modern information ecosystem has made our jobs as healers much harder. It's easy to find books, articles, blogs, YouTube videos, and social media posts encouraging people to increase their fat consumption and blaming carbohydrates for our country's epidemic of metabolic disorders. If eating more fat and cutting carbs to zero were the fastest way to health, then we would have seen a massive epidemic of chronic disease in the 1800s when most people in the United States ate a carb-rich diet. Then we would have seen a miraculous turnaround in the 1900s when the United States transitioned to an industrialized food system and high-fat foods like milk, butter, cheese, and meat became more readily accessible.

Did we see that? Nope.

We saw the exact opposite.

So how is it that our society continues to ignore the role saturated fat plays in its diet? If the evidence against it is so irrefutable, why do so many patients and healers remain confused about what to eat?

Good question. In the next chapter, we'll explore how the food industry uses techniques pioneered by other industries to manipulate science and public opinion to protect their products despite the trouble they bring to public health.

THE PROBLEM WITH LOW-CARB, HIGH-FAT DIET BOOKS

A spate of pseudoscientific diet books in recent years have advocated diets in which people dramatically cut their carbohydrate consumption and increase their fat consumption.

The premise of these books—and the repackaged "keto-genic diet" craze—is that cutting carbs speeds up fat loss and increases calorie burn.

These programs roughly adhere to the Atkins diet first published in 1972, and various versions of low-carb diet books recommend a diet rich in protein and fat and low in carbs. The underlying claim is that under this diet your body switches from burning carbs to burning fat, a process called ketosis. Documentaries like "The Magic Pill" and "Fathead" claim amazing health benefits from this strategy of eating.

Low-carb, high-fat proselytizers like journalists Gary Taubes and Nina Teicholz argue that by reducing your carb calories and replacing them with fat, you drive down insulin levels, boost calorie burn, and melt away fat.

Taubes and Teicholz make a lot of noise and sell a lot of books, but the truth is that this approach has never been scientifically proven. In fact, when researchers from the National Institutes of Health tested the premise in a metabolic ward study funded by Gary Taubes's own group, NuSi, they found no evidence of the dramatic effects promised by these books. In fact, the metabolic ward study reinforced an earlier study by the same scientists that found that cutting fat led to higher body fat loss than cutting carbs.[33]

You can lose weight on a low-carb diet over the short-term, but the benefit wears off after several months.

If Atkins and diets like it were an easy solution to obesity and diabetes, America would have figured that out pretty quickly in the first decade of this century, when 11 percent of Americans were on a low carbohydrate diet.

The claim that low-carb diets improve certain health conditions—such as diabetes, high blood pressure, and cardiovascular disease—is technically true as long as the diet helps you to lose weight. Any diet that helps you lose excessive weight will improve those conditions.

But the American Heart Association, the American College of Cardiology, and the Obesity Society have all concluded that there isn't enough scientific evidence that a low-carb diet provides heart-healthy benefits. In fact, there is plenty of evidence that a high-fat diet will cause a plethora of health problems, particularly if the foods you chose to eat are high in saturated fat.

What's more, many of these books, including *Good Calories, Bad Calories* by Taubes and *Big Fat Surprise* by Teicholz, are based on erroneous assumptions and inaccuracies. Neuroscientist Stephan Guyenet, an expert on obesity, calls Taubes "the single largest source of public misinformation in my area of expertise." Although Taubes and Guyenet agree to a point about refined carbohydrates being fattening, Guyenet objects to the way Taubes rejects the importance of calorie intake and dietary fat intake.

Teicholz, meanwhile, caught flak a few years ago when she attacked the USDA Dietary Guidelines Advisory Committee report. Teicholz's book advises eating more red meat, cheese, butter, and eggs, so when the committee's report said the opposite, she complained publicly. She wrote commentaries in *The New York Times* and the *British Medical Journal*, claiming the committee ignored studies that failed to confirm an association between saturated fats and heart disease. In fact, the committee of scientists and medical professionals considered those studies and still concluded that "reducing saturated fat by reducing and/or modifying dietary fat reduced the risk of cardiovascular events by 17 percent."[34]

People like Taubes and Teicholz write for people who want to believe that high-fat foods are good for them and that saturated fat is harmless. Taubes and Teicholz must defend their flawed reasoning so people will continue to buy their books.

We're not going to go through each of the claims made in these flawed books, but if you did, you'd find that the sources Taubes and Teicholz cite often say exactly the opposite of what the journalists claim they say.[35]

Chapter 2

TROUBLE WITH CHANGE

I'm a big hockey fan. I listen to a regular radio show about my favorite team, and one night the announcer was talking about how he smokes cigarettes. He doesn't see anything wrong with it. He doesn't believe any of the research that shows cigarette smoking causes lung cancer.

This announcer isn't an idiot, and in a broad sense, he's not alone. If he were a nonsmoker looking at the clinical research showing lung damage caused by smoking, he would see the danger and make the decision to never take up cigarettes. But he has a bias—he's already a smoker and seems to enjoy cigarettes—and for that reason, he chooses to believe smoking is not bad for him.

We don't like hearing that our favorite habits can kill us.

My dad was another example of this. He loved cheese omelets, steak, and York Peppermint Patties—three things high in saturated fat. When he developed diabetes, I told him that he had to change his habits. But he didn't change a thing. I was a doctor, I was well educated, and my father trusted me. But he loved high-fat foods, and he wouldn't quit. Consequently, he died of vascular dementia brought on by eating the food he loved.

People in this country have 150 years of behavior patterns built around our industrial food system, which develops delicious products that aren't particularly good for us. Pizza is the number-two source of saturated fat in the typical American diet. There is a pizza parlor on every block and you can get a pizza delivered to your house within a half hour any time you want it.

My patients tell me they never order from Starbucks but there sure seem to be a lot of Starbucks out there.

According to *The New York Times*, Americans eat thirty-three pounds of cheese and cheese products each year, three times what we ate forty years ago and ten times what we did a century ago. Groups like Dairy Management Inc., a dairy farmer trade group, work to increase sales and demand for dairy products through its dairy checkoff program. One way they do this is by working with fast food restaurants on recipes that use more products like cheese. In 2018, for instance, DMI convinced Pizza Hut to add 25 percent more cheese to its pan pizza by convincing the chain that consumers wanted more cheese.[36]

It's true that we love cheese, even though many know that it's rich in saturated fat and that our consumption of it should be strictly limited.

Consider for a moment what would happen if the government told us that Brussels sprouts were bad for our health. Do you think people would triple their consumption of Brussels sprouts the way they did with cheese? What happened when people were getting diarrhea from Romaine lettuce? Did they keep eating it because they love it so much?

But when there is a risk of cancer, heart attack, and stroke from foods like bacon and sausage, people laugh it off. "Oh, you've got to die from something," they'll say.

People are biased toward the habits they love and are deeply reluctant to make changes, even if the change improves their health. We all get into routines, and those habits are difficult to break.

The food industry is aware of this and has engineered

some of its food to make it hard to quit eating. A good example is a Cheeto. You pop one in your mouth, and you get a crunch when you bite down. You chew it briefly, but by the time you swallow, there is almost nothing there. So you grab two more and pop them in your mouth. Before you know it, you've eaten about 500 calories of Cheetos, and you don't feel the least bit full. The food industry's term for this is "vanishing caloric density."[37] The brain is fooled into thinking you haven't consumed any calories and that you're still hungry. Time for dinner!

LET'S CONFUSE OUR CUSTOMERS

In addition to finding new ways to pump us full of cheese, bacon, and gooey cookies, the food industry has found many other slightly devious ways to confuse customers about the actual dangers of some of the industry's offerings.

In her book, *Unsavory Truths*, nutrition expert Marion Nestle (no relation to the Swiss food producer) exposes the food industry's systematic manipulation of the science surrounding food and its related health effects. The industry routinely hires its own researchers and spotlights anomalies from legitimate research in public relations efforts to discredit the overall findings. The goal is not to scientifically prove the benefits of high-fat or unhealthy foods but to merely raise doubts that the legitimate studies are accurate.

This strategy found traction in 2008 when dairy producers and processors from thirty-five countries gathered in Mexico City to discuss how the industry could improve the public's perception of dairy products.

At the time, there was uniform agreement among dietitians, cardiologists, endocrinologists, and cancer researchers that people needed to drastically limit saturated fat in their diets. The problem for the dairy industry was that its products—from milkfat to cheese to butter—were the largest source of saturated fat in the diets of many industrialized nations, including the United States. The industry couldn't continue to grow market share if people were afraid of a key component in so many of their products.

So, according to Martijn Katan, a world-renowned expert on diet and cardiovascular disease who helped document the harm caused by trans fat, the industry set out on a campaign to "neutralize the negative impact of milkfat by regulators and medical professionals."[38]

This was not a campaign to change the science.

In fact, someone conducting a campaign to change science is not a scientist. Scientists don't work that way. Scientists research issues that are unsettled and try to figure out how things work. If the goal were to disprove scientific findings about dietary saturated fat, the first step would have been for researchers to go back over the original experiments to see if they got different results.

This isn't what they did.

In the main articles that tried to change the consensus, all that was done was a reanalysis of old data. Not a single patient had blood drawn. Not a single animal was placed on a high saturated fat diet to show its health improved. Not a single patient was put on a diet high in saturated fat and then examined for changes in their health. In fact, the industry steered away from the appropriate kind of scientific research that would overturn such a bedrock scientific fact, because that kind of research would only show how bad their product truly is.

This is nothing new. In the 1970s, the food industry had an attack dog who also tried to use fallacious statistical arguments and distractions to get people to avoid listening to a scientific consensus, and he was met with a relatively stern rebuke from Ancel Keys, the Harvard-trained physiologist who launched the Seven Countries Study we discussed in chapter 1. Keys stated:

> The question is: Do these saturated fatty acids in the diet cause a rise in serum cholesterol? *That question is no longer debatable.* How the result is brought about will be

known in due course; the question is the subject of intense study in a number of research centers (emphasis mine).[39]

The facts have been certain for more than a half century. So, rather than do the necessary basic science with results so predictable there are multiple equations to describe them, the industry embarked on a PR campaign.

ORCHESTRATING SCIENCE

The dairy industry found statisticians, doctors, and scientists who were made sympathetic to their cause, and these researchers started manipulating old data to obtain findings that suggested there was no definitive evidence that people who ate diets high in saturated fat ran a higher risk of heart disease.

In the primary study that began the media coverage—a meta-analysis or "study of studies"—researchers Ronald Krauss and Patty Siri-Tarino[40] reached the conclusion that there was "insufficient evidence" that saturated fatty acids cause increased risk of cardiovascular disease.

Krauss and Siri-Tarino did this with a trick known as "controlling for a dependent variable."

That is, they controlled for cholesterol levels, which are the main mechanism that causes vascular disease in people who eat diets high in saturated fat. This has the effect of artificially increasing the focus of their studies entirely on a small group of people who by some quirk in their genetics can eat loads of saturated fat and not get an increase in their LDL and Apo(b), the dangerous cholesterol and its carrier protein.

Since saturated fat reliably raises LDL cholesterol in metabolic ward studies,[41] and since the reason saturated fat causes vascular disease is because it raises cholesterol, these researchers were able to magically make the connection between saturated fat and vascular disease go away by discounting the effects of saturated fat in the people it harms the most.

In addition, the study didn't show that saturated fat is good; all they say is that when you make these adjustments, saturated fat is not harmful. Sadly, when people hear that something thought to be dangerous isn't, their natural reaction is to think it is beneficial.

This questionable approach would be like doing a study on the relationship between cigarettes and lung cancer and controlling for lighters and matches. Everyone in the study carries around cigarettes, but only a portion of that group actually smokes their cigarettes. By controlling for lighters and matches, you wash out the 99.9 percent of people who both carry cigarettes and smoke them, and you elevate the importance of those who carry cigarettes but don't smoke them. This allows you to conclude that cigarettes aren't related to lung cancer at all once you control for lighters and matches. This is what's known as overcontrolling or overadjusting the data to reach a conclusion that supports your preconceived notion.

So this wasn't an attempt to overturn a century of research into saturated fat. It was an attempt to get headlines. The National Dairy Council-funded "research" was faulty and was attacked by the science community. But that didn't bother dairy industry leaders because they weren't interested in altering the science in the first place. They wanted to create doubt, and they needed help from the media.

They got it.

HOW THE MEDIA HELP

After this study came out, the media latched on to the controversy and started running stories like the cover of *Time* magazine that said, "Eat Butter. Scientists labeled fat the enemy. Why they were wrong."

The media love this type of story much more than a story that reinforces something we already know. If someone wants to write a story about how seatbelts are a good thing, the newspaper isn't interested. Everybody knows that seatbelts are good. But if someone calls the newspaper and says they want to write a story that seatbelts are bad because they kill people, the newspaper is clearing space on page one for it.

When it comes to saturated fat, people were tired of hearing how it was bad for their health and caused heart disease, since they had continued to eat large amounts of it even in the face of public announcements that it led to heart disease. The public had grown tired of hearing that for over half a century. But here were a couple of scientists saying bacon, beef, and butter are good for you by saying it wasn't bad for you! (They said it wasn't bad so people thought it was good.)

That's news!

For the food industry, this kind of media coverage is as good as those high-fat "bliss" foods it sells its hungry customers. You get the picture of the eggs scrambled in butter, the piled-high burger, or that overflowing milkshake, and you get the headline that says it's okay to eat eggs, beef, and ice cream again. Most readers will only see that and head off to enjoy their old pleasures again. They have other things to do with their day. When someone tells you your wife is beautiful or your kids are smart, you don't investigate it much. Instead, people generally look for stories that confirm what they wish the world were like.

And the real scientists get drowned out and relegated to writing letters to obscure academic journals.

In 2014, a study from Cambridge University replicated the Krauss and Siri-Tarino analysis and found no evidence that eating saturated fat increased heart disease. The study from Dr. Rajiv Chowdhury concluded that arteries are not clogged by saturated fat but by an excess of sugary foods and carbohydrates, and stories about the findings appeared in media around the world. *The New York Times* story[42] that went out to the paper's 2.2 million subscribers was accompanied by a large photo of a bacon cheeseburger with a fried-egg topping.

Unfortunately, the story about how several respected researchers thoroughly discredited Chowdhury's study did not get the same kind of play.

The Department of Nutrition at Harvard School of Public Health's criticism that the study is "seriously misleading" and "contains major errors and omissions" and "should be disregarded" ran in the comments section of *Annals of Internal Medicine*, which goes out to about 150,000 people.[43]

I wonder which message got through to the public?

DIETARY FAT AND DÉJÀ VU: HOW THE BATTLE OVER TRANS FATS RESEMBLES TODAY'S FIGHT OVER SATURATED FATS[44]

Artificial trans fat was introduced in the 1950s as a healthy alternative to animal-based saturated fats. At the time, health advocates strongly urged Americans to remove saturated fats, such as in butter and beef, from their diets, and trans fats were touted as a healthy alternative.

The new artificial fat was created by adding hydrogen to natural vegetable oil (a process known as hydrogenation), and was used for decades in margarine, Crisco, and a wide variety of processed foods. It was cheap to make, tasted good, and increased the shelf life of certain products.

By the 1980s, however, researchers were finding strong evidence that trans fats contributed to diabetes and heart disease. Researchers found alarming build-ups of trans fatty acids in the arteries of heart-attack victims. Studies on pigs showed the same frightening build-up of plaque and heart disease.

In the face of this, the food industry, led by Kraft and Proctor & Gamble, hired researchers to refute the damaging trans fat findings (sound familiar?) and discourage more research into the dangers posed by artificial trans fat.

People like Walter Willett of Harvard, who in 1980 started tracking 100,000 women and found an alarming increase in heart disease risk among those who ate food with artificial trans fat, had trouble getting papers published. Willett finally published his results in 1993, but it would be another twenty-five years before trans fats were banned.

In 2015, thirty-five years after researchers discovered the troubling health effects from trans fats, the FDA finally ruled trans fats unsafe. It was another three years before trans fats were formally banned.[45]

Ironically, artificial trans fats have been banned while saturated fats—the unhealthy component trans fats were designed to replace—remain a big part of the American diet. The molecular structure of trans fats is almost identical to saturated fat (only one hydrogen atom is different), and both fats produce the same health effects—clogged arteries, obesity, diabetes, and all the metabolic ailments that come with them.

STICK TO THE SCIENCE

It's a well-established scientific fact that dietary saturated fat increases a person's dangerous LDL cholesterol level and that elevated LDL levels increase the risk of vascular disease, strokes, heart attacks, and other ailments.

Scientists don't debate these facts, but low-carb gurus, bloggers, and internet "journalists" do.

Nevertheless, the effort to confuse the public about saturated fat, which started in the late 1990s and ramped up after the dairy industry's Mexico City conference, continues to this day. Here's the page from the food industry's playbook:

- You find a scientist willing to say saturated fat is not that harmful. It helps if that scientist has an opposing theory, such as that carbohydrates and not saturated fat cause heart disease.
- You get that scientist to cherry-pick enough of the findings from legitimate scientific studies to support their contrary position. The scientist publishes a paper that says that saturated fats aren't that bad.
- You get media attention because this finding is controversial and interesting! You mean it's okay to eat bacon and eggs again? People will click on this and share it.
- The word gets around and now all those people who really don't want to make changes to their diet have an excuse to continue eating poorly. They aren't really doing nutrition research anyway.

The authors of these phony studies aren't trying to add to the scientific record or change the minds of scientists.

When it comes to the dangers of saturated fat, most scientists can't have their minds changed because the factual record showing the dangers of saturated fat is too strong. Instead of doing new research, the purpose of these deliberately obfuscatory studies from people like Krauss, Siri-Tarino, and Chowdhury is to create headlines.

Most of us and our patients likely don't have the time or knowledge to tear apart a study like Chowdhury's or Krauss and Siri-Tarino's the way the Harvard scientists did.[46] So as medical practitioners, we have to make sure our message is clear and irrefutable: if you replace saturated fat in your diet with refined grains and sugar—the largest source of calories in the United States diet—your risk of heart disease remains relatively high. But if you replace those saturated fats with starch from whole grains, whole potatoes or sweet potatoes, whole beans, poly-unsaturated fat, or monounsaturated fat in the form of olives, nuts, or other higher-fat plant foods, your risk of heart disease is significantly reduced.

If your patients still seem unconvinced, pull back even further and offer this overarching perspective: among people who have low LDL (dangerous cholesterol) but don't exercise at all, heart disease is rare. Among people who have low LDLs but have other risk factors, such as high blood pressure, heart disease is still rare. But among people who don't smoke, don't have high blood pressure, exercise regularly, but have very high LDLs, heart disease is common. Other than powerful drugs, the most effective way to lower LDL is to cut saturated fat and cholesterol from your diet.[47]

PURE STUDY NOT SO PURE

In 2017, researchers published the results of the Prospective Urban Rural Epidemiology study, which followed the diets of more than 135,000 people in eighteen countries across five continents for seven years.[48] They found that those who consumed the most dietary fat (35 percent of their daily calories) were 23 percent less likely to die than those with the lowest fat intake (only 10 percent of their daily calories). What's more, those with the highest consumption of carbohydrates (77 percent of their daily calories) were 28 percent more likely to have died than those whose diet was only 46 percent carbohydrates.

The authors of the study, which was funded by pharmaceutical companies, performed a neat trick, much like the one conducted by the Siri-Tarino and Choudhry meta-analyses. While reviewing the data for cardiovascular disease, they excluded all people in the studies who had established heart disease, removing the people most likely to die of cardiovascular disease. Yet they included all deaths from things like HIV and traumatic deaths from tsunamis. The study concluded that a high carbohydrate diet was more likely to kill you than a diet low in carbohydrates and that "total fat and individual types of fat were related to lower total mortality," but left out the fact that many of the deaths were deaths in Zimbabwe from the HIV epidemic and deaths in India from the tsunami that struck there in 2004.

I don't know about you, but I am pretty sure the fat/carbohydrate ratio of the diet doesn't really play much into those deaths. If your goal is finding out the effects of diet on health, it would strike me as valuable to exclude those deaths as well. Since Canadians and Swedes face very low risk from HIV and tidal waves, this really helped the stats for high-fat diets, when added to the exclusion of anyone with heart problems at the beginning of the study.

The headlines over stories about the study were, in the view of the Harvard School of Public Health, "sensational."[49] The media said things like, *Study Challenges Conventional Wisdom on Fats, Fruits, and Vegetables*, and *PURE Shakes Up Nutritional Field*, and *Huge New Study Casts Doubt on Conventional Wisdom About Fat and Carbs*.

The scientists at Harvard and elsewhere found several problems with the study, including:

· This analysis of the PURE data oversimplified what constituted a carbohydrate, making no distinction between diets high in sugar and refined ingredients and diets high in healthier whole plant foods, such as fruits, vegetables, legumes, and whole grains. In fact, another paper published using the PURE data showed that diets high in unprocessed plant foods markedly lowered overall mortality. Sugary, refined foods can lead to type 2 diabetes, heart disease, obesity, macular degeneration, ovulatory infertility, and colorectal cancer, while complex carbohydrates help control type 2 diabetes and improve weight loss.[50]

· The PURE study didn't factor in the effects of the "poverty diet" many of the study's participants consumed, so the health problems related to a high-carb diet were likely to have actually been the result of poverty and poor nutrition.

· A team of doctors writing a commentary in the American Journal of Medicine noted that the recent influx of highly processed, high-carb foods triggering sharp jumps in cases of diabetes, obesity, and heart disease in places like Brazil and India can't be compared to saturated fat. "...the question of whether processed carbohydrates or saturated fats are worse for cardiovascular health does not warrant scientific evaluation because we have adequate evidence to indicate that both are harmful (and likely so) and should be limited, if not eliminated from the diet," the doctors wrote.

Again, if your patients are just looking at the news headlines, they would think saturated fat is good for them. Your patients are probably not reading the scientific journals where legitimate doctors and scientists refute these findings. In this sense, the ongoing PURE study follows the same pattern as its food-industry-serving predecessors: generate headlines, overcomplicate the science, and give people an excuse to continue eating pizza, fries, and ice cream.

THE WONDERFUL DAIRY INDUSTRY

How does the food industry get away with these shenanigans? For the dairy industry, it's easy to see how: dairy producers have a century of propaganda that milk is good for everybody and everyone should drink it. Their product is pure sweetness and light and comes from these wonderful happy cows living on bucolic grass-hay dairy farms where the animals stroll in once a day to lovingly surrender their beautiful milk for the people. You rarely see actual footage of a dairy in full operation because that would be unappetizing, especially if they show what happens to the male calves born and quickly slaughtered for veal.

If the dairy industry were interested in proving that butter, cream, high-fat milk, and cheese are safe and wholesome, they would simply fund a study where you take healthy people, feed them more saturated fat, and show how their health improved.

But they don't do that.

Instead, they do the same thing the tobacco industry did when it was trying to hide the fact that its products killed people. Faced with mounting evidence that smoking was harmful, the tobacco industry used sophisticated public relations to weaken and distort the emerging science. The tobacco industry never took nonsmokers, made them smoke, and then showed that their lungs got better, even though they made that claim earlier in the twentieth century. The tobacco industry knew they wouldn't get that result and never bothered to try. The food industry is following the same playbook.

Any study will have some kinks—minor things that don't look normal. That's how science works. And it's good that people can look at the same set of facts and draw slightly different conclusions. That paves the way for future studies and a refined view of the bigger picture. But when you compare the mountain of evidence that saturated fat is bad for you to the evidence that it's either neutral or good for you, it's like comparing Mount Everest to a gopher mound.[51]

With that in mind, let's move on and look at what science tells us about the physical damage caused by too much saturated fat.

Chapter 3

A DANGEROUS MEAL

Actor James Gandolfini was vacationing in Italy in June 2013 with his thirteen-year-old son, and after a day visiting the Vatican and seeing the sights, the two sat down for a meal at the Boscolo Exedra Roma hotel's outdoor restaurant.

Gandolfini was known as a man of big appetites, and that was on display this night.[52] The *Sopranos* star ate two orders of fried prawns with mayonnaise chili sauce and a large order of foie gras. He also had a few piña coladas, rum chasers, and beer. All told, his meal amounted to 2,730 calories and was dripping in saturated fat. The foie gras alone had more saturated fat than a person should eat in a single day, and Gandolfini was just getting started.

There was also cream in the piña coladas and gobs of saturated fat in the fried prawns and mayonnaise.

Three hours after the meal, the fifty-one-year-old actor was dead of a heart attack.

While tragic, Gandolfini's death was a predictable event for people who have a high-fat diet and then sit down for a blockbuster meal glistening with more saturated fat. When people eat a high-saturated-fat meal, their existing arterial plaque can begin to form cholesterol crystals that can slice open the inner lining (endothelium) of one of their coronary arteries.[53] This creates a blood clot that blocks the flow of blood to the heart muscle, creating a rhythm disturbance and sometimes making the heart fibrillate.

This is a heart attack.

People in this situation suddenly can't get blood and oxygen to the rest of their body, including their brain, and they die. If they're lucky and someone is nearby with some paddles to shock their heart and give them cardiopulmonary resuscitation, they might recover. But if they're alone in their hotel room like Gandolfini was, their chances of living are slim.

In fact, for one in four men in the United States with heart disease, their first symptom of the problem is when they die of a heart attack. The first time they become aware of a problem is during those moments between starting to feel bad and then falling over dead. In women, the ratio is worse: one in three with heart disease won't show any symptoms until they suffer a heart attack and die. Heart attacks like these are more common on Christmas and New Year's when people tend to overindulge on rich food.[54]

HEALTH RISKS FROM SATURATED FAT

Cardiovascular disease is the leading cause of death worldwide, and that is what respected organizations like the American Heart Association focus on when they recommend people reduce saturated fat. Reducing our intake of saturated fat would save hundreds of thousands of lives each year globally by reducing the number of heart attacks, strokes, and cases of congestive heart failure.

But reducing dietary saturated fat would also go a long way toward improving the overall well-being of many millions more, reducing their risk of a host of related ailments ranging from the deadly to the merely annoying.

In addition to the common cardiovascular issues caused by weakened blood flow to heart and brain, patients consuming too much saturated fat can also suffer from diabetes,[55] dementia,[56] [57] hearing loss,[58] lower back pain,[59] erectile dysfunction,[55] and weakened connective tissue.[60] People develop fatty liver, which brings on digestive issues, nausea, and acid reflux.[61] These people also struggle to stay awake after lunch or battle general fatigue during the day. Overall, it's hard to imagine anyone on a high-saturated-fat diet thriving through the length of their lifespan.

Take Shawn Baker, for example. This orthopedic surgeon went on a diet composed entirely of meat. He had been doing it for two years, and had blood tests done. His cholesterol was very high, and his testosterone level was very low. His blood sugar was also in the prediabetic range, even though he was eating essentially zero carbohydrates.[62]

Why is fat causing all these diseases and problems? The best way to understand these widespread and sometimes debilitating effects is to look at what happens to your blood when you have a steady diet of food rich in fat.

A LOOK AT THE BLOOD

The effect of saturated fat on vascular disease is well documented in countless studies dating back more than a century. Experiments have shown how the arteries in people who eat a single fatty meal are unable to dilate adequately to allow blood to flow around a clot. Restricted dilation can persist for up to twelve hours.[63]

At the same time, a person's blood serum after a fatty meal can become milky because it's so full of fat. Healthy serum is clear with a yellowish tint, but serum from someone whose regular diet is rich in any type of fat will be creamy yellow, opaque, and thick—cloudy from all that fat in it. Your blood has a hard time finding a place to remove that fat because the body can only excrete or metabolize tiny amounts of it. Your blood flow slows way down and gets sluggish as it deposits that fatty stuff along the walls of your arteries.

We call that creamy liquid lipemic serum. Not every person with cardiovascular disease has it; you can still have serious problems even if your serum is not lipemic. Lipemia is just the worst-case scenario.

When I was in college working as a phlebotomist at St. Helena Hospital in California, I drew blood from many people who were entering the hospital's McDougall Program, run by Dr. John McDougall, MD. In anticipation of that program, which emphasized a healthy, low-fat diet, these patients would often stop off on their way to the hospital for one last blow-out meal at a fast food restaurant.

I would see lipemic serum all the time. Not surprisingly, the plaque that builds up in your arteries is the same creamy yellow as that lipemic serum. If you compare the chemical components of the fats in your blood with the plaque in your arteries, you'll find they are quite similar.

This process of blood serum turning milky and then depositing the fat along the arterial wall is more predictable than rain. Tell me what you last ate and I can predict whether your serum will have that waxy sheen to it.[64] When someone suggests that a diet high in saturated fat is somehow good for you—that "butter is back" and you could eat as much cheese and cream as you'd like—you should take the advice as seriously as you would dating advice from Ariana Grande. The only way these claims about the benefits of saturated fat make sense is if you're looking for any excuse to put bacon on your donuts and cheese sauce on your broccoli.

I explain this process of lipemic serum to my patients by asking them if they ever eat beets or asparagus. When you eat beets, you get this moment later in the bathroom when you look down at your pee and you think, *"Am I dying?"*

Then you recall the beets. The pigment in the beets is absorbed from your gastrointestinal tract and circulated by your blood. Then it's removed by your kidneys and siphoned into your urine. The same thing happens when you get that odor in your pee from asparagus.

BLOOD TURNS TO SLUDGE

Something similar happens when you dip your bread into that big hunk of brie. The fat from the cheese (most cheese is 75 percent saturated fat) circulates in your blood. But unlike the beet pigment, the fat has nowhere to go. You can't pee it out.

Instead, the blood becomes more viscous, and this allows the blood to clot more easily. In many cases, the artery will sense this and dilate 20 percent to allow the blood to flow around the clot. When this happens, you don't typically even notice a problem. However, when a high-saturated-fat meal has reduced your arteries' ability to dilate, you are more likely to get a clot that blocks your blood flow and kills you.[65] Those folks lolling around on the couch after their Thanksgiving meal aren't sleepy from tryptophan; they're groggy from sludgy blood. They are sleepy because their blood isn't delivering enough oxygen to tissues that need it.

The results of routine consumption of high-fat meals, particularly those that are also sugary, are stark and easy to discern. Arterial plaque develops. The blood becomes thick and slow-moving. Rigid arteries are unable to expand. And finally, your single, high-fat meal increases the blood's fibrinogen, the clotting protein, which allows clots to form more quickly and causes the blood to flow in a Rouleaux formation—stacks of red blood cells that stick together and form a kind of languid train that struggles to flow through your body.[66]

Researchers have filmed the process, showing the blood surging through an artery before the big meal and then slowing down as the red blood cells adhere to each other and then stack up after the high-fat meal is consumed. The formation can't fit into your capillaries, which can take just one red blood cell at a time. You see the same kind of torpid blood flow in patients with serious health problems, such as infections, multiple myeloma, connective tissue disorders, diabetes, and cancers.

That deadly sequence of saturated fat forming plaque and creating a cholesterol crystal that tears the epithelium is commonplace in any society with an industrialized food system and diets rich in saturated fat. Excluding traumatic injuries, these medical emergencies are the most common life-threatening events seen in emergency and operating rooms.

IT'S ALL WELL DOCUMENTED

The lipemia can come from any type of fat, but the body's

way of dealing with excessive saturated fat is particularly troublesome.

The body stores excess saturated fat in the organs and linings of the abdominal cavity, which is the worst possible place for it. Storing the fat there leads to the development of metabolic syndrome, which is a group of risk factors, including high blood pressure, high blood sugar, unhealthy lipid levels, and the abdominal fat itself.

It's not just beer that gives you a "beer belly." Let's call it a "butter belly."

Not surprisingly, nearly 50 million Americans have metabolic syndrome—one in six. The most significant risk factor for atherosclerotic heart disease is diabetes, and we'll talk in a later chapter about how saturated fat has been implicated in the development of that disease.

We'll also touch later on dementia, so, for now, we'll just say that patients with Alzheimer's often have a massive amount of plaque in their arteries. An Alzheimer's-diseased brain shrinks due to inadequate blood flow, and we have evidence that Alzheimer's is related to atherosclerosis and dietary intake of saturated fat.

All told, saturated fat contributes independently—separate from its effect on cholesterol—to five different mechanisms that create heart attacks and strokes, causing inflammation,[67] blood clotting,[68] slowed blood flow,[69] less vessel dilation,[70] and bacterial toxins[71] circulating in the blood.

As we've mentioned before, we are just scratching the surface when it comes to describing the damage caused to the human body from excessive dietary saturated fat. We would need an 800-page book to go into detail about all the harmful effects, but the ones we mention here should give your patients plenty of reasons to find ways to limit their consumption of saturated fat.

Despite the thousands who die each year from cardiovascular disease, most people's bodies are able to adjust to their owner's unhealthy habits for a prolonged period. It's not a great *quality* of life—they're tired and sick and possibly increasingly confused—but at least these people are alive.

And they can do something to get better.

GETTING TO ZERO

Whether you're a healthcare professional or a patient reading this book, you should know that trying to reduce your saturated fat intake to zero is nearly impossible. Saturated fat is in a lot of good foods in small quantities, so even if you try to eliminate it completely, you're probably still getting 1 to 2 percent of your calories from saturated fat. Also, if you eat more calories than you burn up through activity, your body, just like a cow's does, can make its own saturated fat.

In 2017, the heart association's Presidential Advisory on Dietary Fats and CVD recommended all patients keep their saturated fat to no more than 10 percent of all the calories they consume. The group noted that the average consumption of saturated fat in the United States is nearly 12 percent, and that fewer than one in three Americans keep their consumption below 10 percent. Patients who already have elevated levels of the dangerous LDL cholesterol should keep their consumption down to 5–6 percent, the advisory panel said, and it recommended a diet high in whole plant foods, grains, tubers, legumes, fruits, and vegetables.

Although the AHA has been recommending reducing dietary saturated fat since 1961 (nearly sixty years) the advisory panel nevertheless reviewed multiple randomized clinical trials, meta-analyses, prospective observational studies, and animal studies to reach these conclusions. This was not a cursory review designed to garner headlines, and unfortunately it didn't get much media attention—except when someone wanted to defend butter, steak, and coconut oil.

Why are these clear, well-documented recommendations so often overlooked? Probably because the sheer enormity of what the AHA is saying is difficult for people to fully grasp.

Only when you comprehend just how damaging saturated fat is and how prevalent it is in the typical Western diet, does it become clear how significantly our patients have to change if they want to avoid these noncommunicable diseases or reverse their effects. As healthcare professionals, we are asking them to make sweeping changes to their diet. It's a big ask. There will be a lot of confused, awkward silences in those exam rooms as patients try to absorb what we're telling them. But we have to tell them and we have to acknowledge that what we're asking them to do is not simple or easy. Only then will they begin to comprehend how dramatically their behavior must change.

Here's an example of a fictional medical crisis that is on the same order as saturated fat. Say science revealed a widespread disease caused by wearing pants. Many of us have been wearing pants since we were young children, and now we are learning that they are threatening our health and our doctors are advising us to stop wearing pants.

Remember: this is hypothetical. But imagine how shocking it would be to have to stop wearing pants. Patients would feel weird not wearing pants anymore. They would probably look around them and see a lot of people still wearing pants—despite the warnings about the disease caused by pants—and as a result our patients would have even more trouble changing. What's more, those from the healthcare profession advising people to don kilts or loincloths and stop wearing pants would no doubt be ridiculed.

Yet, for the purposes of our illustration, the fact remains: wearing pants increases your risk of getting horrible diseases that afflict millions of people.

In that light, a kilt or a silk-brocade loincloth wouldn't sound so ridiculous. Doesn't a dramatic wardrobe change make sense if it cuts down on your risk of dying or becoming desperately sick from wearing pants? Of course it does! But many people would insist on continuing to wear pants.

When it comes to saturated fat, we're up against a similar challenge. People love cheese and ice cream and hamburgers and French fries as much as they love their Levi's and Gap jeans. They've enjoyed these foods all their lives. And now someone is telling them to stop?

Yes, someone *is* telling them to stop. You are. Because

if your patient thinks it will be a big inconvenience to have to cut fast food or pizza out of their diet, urge them to consider how inconvenient the heart attacks, strokes, dementia, or diabetes caused by their diet will be.

I'm not advocating a "tough-love" approach with your patients, but I *am* advocating that you acknowledge the scope of the changes you're asking them to make. Be frank with them.

Changing your diet *dramatically* is hard to do. But if you want to live a better, longer life, this is what you'll have to do.

WHEN HEALTH ADVICE IS BAD FOR BUSINESS

One critic of the AHA advisory came from a website that sells coconut oil and coconut-oil diet books. Ironically, that website, Sustainable Dish, argued that the AHA cherrypicked its data to support its conclusions and that the organization was corrupted by corporate influence. Journalist Nina Teicholz, the author of *Big Fat Surprise: Why Butter, Meat and Cheese Belong in a Healthy Diet* who also has a side gig lobbying for the beef industry to make USDA dietary guidelines more beef-friendly, criticized the heart association in the *Los Angeles Times*, claiming the advisory was the product of "longstanding bias." That bias is apparently the result of a hundred years of scientific research clearly showing saturated fat is bad.

Now, you can understand why someone who gets commissions on the sale of coconut-oil diet books or books extolling the benefits of butter, cheese, and meat might have an inherent bias. But what does the AHA panel—a group of scientists from Harvard, Tufts, Johns Hopkins, and the New York University School of Medicine—have to gain by warning people about saturated fat? Are they getting a commission on broccoli sales?

The key takeaway here is this: if your patients are willing to do the hard work it takes to reduce their saturated fat calories and replace them with better foods, they can make massive changes in their long-term health outcomes. They may live longer, and the quality of their lives is improved.

Even after years of eating high-saturated-fat meals and developing arterial plaque, patients who change their diet and eliminate saturated fat will get better. You can't fully remove plaque once it's there, but studies suggest you can shrink it by lowering the LDL in your blood and taking statin drugs. The plaque becomes metabolically inactive and then becomes relatively safe. The endothelium over that inactive atherosclerosis will be thick and unlikely to be sliced open.

In severe emergencies, of course, doctors use invasive procedures, such as angiography, angioplasty, stenting, or bypass surgery, to clear away artery-blocking plaques.

A WORD ABOUT OILS

When patients attempt to replace saturated fat in their diet with healthier fats, they should understand that even healthy oils like olive oil—a staple of the Mediterranean diet—have a certain amount of saturated fat in them.

For example, even canola oil, considered the healthiest of the dietary oils, has one gram of saturated fat in each tablespoon. Sunflower oil has 1.4 grams per tablespoon and olive oil has near two grams of saturated fat per tablespoon. Coconut oil, at the other end of the spectrum, has almost 12 grams of saturated fat in every tablespoon. The next-highest concentration of saturated fat among the oils is palm kernel oil, which has just over 11 grams of saturated fat.

Here's a list of some common oils and their saturated fat amounts:

- Canola oil (1 gram/tablespoon)
- Safflower oil (1g/Tbs.)
- Almond oil (1.1g/Tbs.)

- Walnut oil (1.2g/Tbs.)
- Flaxseed oil (1.3g/TBs.)
- Corn oil (1.8g/Tbs.)
- Peanut oil (2.3g/Tbs.)
- Butter (7.3g/Tbs.)

Just because an oil is low in saturated fat isn't a license to use it wantonly. If you give up three tablespoons of coconut oil and start using 18 tablespoons of olive oil, you're getting the same level of saturated fat.

What's a good formula for determining how much to restrict your saturated fat intake? The math is pretty simple. If you eat 2,000 calories a day and you want to limit saturated fat to 10 percent of that amount (the latest USDA Dietary Guidelines for America recommendation), that means you should eat no more than 200 calories, or about 22 grams, of saturated fat.

I think that percentage is too high, however. The AHA recommends keeping your saturated fats to 6 percent or below if you are at risk of heart disease, which everyone is since it's the number-one killer. That would make that 2,000-calorie-a-day target 140 calories, or about 15.4 grams.

Many different types of food have saturated fat occurring naturally in them. Even oatmeal, a food proven to lower cholesterol, has some saturated fat (about .5 grams per single serving) in it. That's because whole-grain oats still have the oil-rich bran and germ in them.

However, because of these foods that naturally have saturated fat, I recommend people aim to reduce their intake of added oils and saturated fat to nothing. Taking that approach helps ensure you are keeping your intake low and it also eliminates the need to keep a calculator handy when you walk into the pantry.

Chapter 4

MANAGING CHOLESTEROL

I saw a patient recently who came in with chest pains. He was a slender man in his late sixties with a family history of high cholesterol. When we tested his blood, his total cholesterol level was 1,100 mg/dL. In medicine, we consider anything over 200 to be high, and anything over 300 is wildly high. He was almost four times higher than that. His LDL, or dangerous cholesterol, was 600 mg/dL with a high normal of 130.

Luckily he'd never had a heart attack or stroke. But angina was a severe problem. He couldn't make it up a flight of stairs without experiencing chest pains. He was eating a standard American diet that included meat, dairy products, and plenty of saturated fat, and although he had

been to a cardiologist and knew about his high cholesterol, he hadn't made any therapeutic lifestyle changes
that would reduce it.

With our help, he made massive changes to his diet. He
went on an almost perfect, plant-based diet, and within
two weeks, his chest pains had eased and his cholesterol
was down to 197—still high, but a vast improvement.
After four weeks, the chest pains all but disappeared. He
could climb the stairs and go shopping at the mall without
having to sit down to rest continually.

We also got him started on a statin drug because, in a
case like this, it's all hands on deck. Within a short time,
his total cholesterol was down to ninety-seven and his
dangerous LDL cholesterol was down to thirty. He still
had massive amounts of plaque in his arterial tree all
through his body, but we knew that since he had reversed
the direction of that plaque growth that he would soon
overcome a lot of the physical limitations caused by the
plaque and the reduced blood flow related to it.

I tell this story to illustrate not only how dangerous high
levels of LDL cholesterol can be but also how quickly lifestyle changes can reduce those LDL cholesterol levels
and ease the functional ills associated with high cholesterol, including lower back pain and erectile dysfunction.
In my office, when people have dangerous levels of LDL

but change their habits and bring it down quickly, they get better within weeks.

THE TRUTH ABOUT CHOLESTEROL

If you ever made rock candy as a kid, then you know that dangling a string into plain water did not produce any rock candy. However, if there was a lot of sugar dissolved in the water, it would latch onto the string and form the crystals.

Cholesterol in your blood makes crystals in the same way. Once you develop plaque in the artery's walls, crystals can form when your blood is high in cholesterol. Those crystals can then slice the inner lining of an artery. A blood clot forms, and if that artery is leading to your heart or your brain, you could suffer a stroke or a heart attack. This is why it is so critical to keep cholesterol levels low because at low levels the crystals don't form.

LDL cholesterol and its carrier protein, Apo(b), are the primary causes of heart and vascular diseases.[72] Respected medical authorities such as the American Heart Association warn that high blood cholesterol should be a concern for anyone, regardless of their age. As people get older, they tend to produce more cholesterol, including total cholesterol and the dangerous LDL. Healthy adults should have their cholesterol checked every four to six years.

The recommendations for cholesterol levels have been dropping for many years. For instance, in the 1950s, Nathan Pritikin had a total cholesterol reading of 300 and was told that was normal. Lucky for him, he felt that number was too high and found ways to bring down his cholesterol through diet and exercise.

Likewise, many doctors today believe the recommended LDL level of 100 is still way too high. In a study published in the Journal of the American College of Cardiology, researchers found that about half of the heart attacks in the US strike people who have an LDL between 100 and 115 and that about 10 to 12 percent of the heart attacks occur in people with an LDL between 70 and 100. That means the majority of heart attacks strike people who have LDL levels that, while dangerous, are considered normal by the current standards. However, the heart attack risk almost disappears in people whose LDL is below 70.[73]

Optimal LDL is 50–70, researchers found. If you've already had a heart attack, you may need to get your LDL down below 50 to reverse the damage.

This dangerous LDL cholesterol is a waxy, fat-like substance that gets deposited in arterial walls, cutting down blood flow. LDL cholesterol is the main source of artery-clogging plaque. Although the average LDL level in the

US has decreased from 123 in 1999–2000 to 111 in 2013–2014[74] (thanks to statin drugs and the US ban on trans fats in foods), that "statistically normal" LDL level of 111 will still cause disease in a high percentage of patients. In fact, each year more than 2 million Americans experience cardiovascular events that account for about 25 percent of all inpatient hospital costs.[75]

That's a big problem, made more worrisome because so much of that pain, suffering, and expense is preventable. Controlling LDL substantially reduces cardiovascular disease morbidity and mortality, and one of the best ways to control LDL levels is with a diet low in saturated fat.[76]

According to the European Atherosclerosis Society, atherosclerotic vascular diseases such as myocardial infarction and ischemic stroke are the leading cause of injury and death throughout the world.[77] It used to be just developed countries had this problem, but the trouble has spread to the entire world as a result of people eating too much saturated fat from tropical oils, animal meats, eggs, fish, and dairy products.

Nevertheless, there are still doctors out there who argue that heart disease is caused by inflammation, not cholesterol. They are a tiny subset of fringe doctors, none of whom are certified lipidologists. None of them has a research program demonstrating the benefits of saturated fat or the benefits of high serum cholesterol, yet they claim both of these things are good for you. This is a tell, a sign that their primary goal is to create media reports and not to change science. If they were able to show that butter was good for any organism, they would have no problem getting that research published. But they never do that kind of research.

Despite this lack of science, every time a member of The International Network of Cholesterol Skeptics (THINCS)[78] publishes something that suggests cholesterol dangers are exaggerated, the media lap it up. *Here's a doctor saying cholesterol isn't important!* Never mind that these wild claims have no scientific backing and that thousands of studies have shown that high cholesterol can kill you.

In the face of claims to the contrary, the EAS in 2017 published a consensus panel statement stating that LDL cholesterol *unquestionably* causes cardiovascular disease.[79] The society felt a consensus statement would help eliminate the confusion among doctors and the public about this huge problem and emphasize the strength of this association between LDL cholesterol and cardiovascular disease. The EAS hoped this would allow healthcare providers to quit wasting time debating the issue and focus instead on helping the millions of people who should change their lifestyle or get the medicine they need to lower LDL.

Yet, the debate continues. In April 2019, when Dr. Aseem Malhotra announced on Twitter a lecture he was giving on "the great cholesterol and statin con," Dr. Michael V. Holmes, a cardiovascular epidemiologist with the Nuffield Department of Population Health at Oxford University, called Malhotra's position "the very antithesis of evidence-based medicine" that is "on a theoretical par with flat-Earthers."[80]

Those of us who treat patients with cardiovascular disease already understand how important it is to get our patients' LDL cholesterol down. When we reduce those levels—either through diet, exercise, drugs, surgery, or all of these treatments—phenomenal results occur. Heart disease is reversed. Our patients' risk of death from all causes drops, mostly by reducing cardiovascular death, the top cause of mortality.[81]

FINDING THE RIGHT LEVEL

To get a sense of where your patients' LDL cholesterol should be, look at nature. A newborn human baby has an LDL between 20 and 40 milligrams per deciliter. Most animals living in the wild have levels from 60 to 80 mg/dL. Almost no organism on Earth spends a substantial amount of time with an LDL over 100.[82] [83] Modern humans with a Western-style diet are the exception. The average LDL cholesterol level among adults in the

United States (111 mg/dL[84]) is well above the healthy LDL cholesterol level of 100 set by the Centers for Disease Control and Prevention.[85]

Some people have genes that drive up their LDL cholesterol levels. One particularly serious genetic condition is called familial hyperlipidemia (FH). People with severe FH inherit two dysfunctional genes—one from each parent—and those genes prevent LDL receptors in the liver from doing their job of keeping cholesterol levels under control. FH patients are at high risk of heart and vascular disease uncommonly early in life.

At the other end of the spectrum are people with familial hypobetalipoproteinemia (FHBL).[86] This condition restricts the body's ability to absorb and transport fats, and this results in patients with low levels of cholesterol in their blood. That may sound like a good thing, but it sometimes isn't; people with a severe case of FHBL can have an abnormal buildup of fats in the liver and can develop fatty liver or cirrhosis.

Regardless of whether your patient's LDL levels are due to genetics or lifestyle, a higher average LDL cholesterol increases their risk of heart disease and allows heart disease to develop earlier in life. For example, people with severe FH begin getting heart attacks in their twenties and thirties. The treatment for FH is the same as for someone with high cholesterol—a low-fat diet, exercise, and cholesterol-lowering drugs. In severe cases, we combine several strong cholesterol-lowering drugs and even filter patients' blood to remove the excess LDL.

Although those cases are rare—between 1 in 500 and 1 in 1,000 people have a severe form of FH[87]—genes nevertheless play a more significant role in LDL than we previously thought. Patients can have one dominant gene that gives them FH, but other patients can also have less-dominant, single-switch genes that affect their cholesterol—although not as much as that one dominant gene. It takes many of those polygenic genes to equal the impact of the single dominant gene that gives you FH.

Here's how I explain it to my patients:

Say you put a boulder in a wheelbarrow. That boulder represents severe high cholesterol from a single genetic cause, and it makes the wheelbarrow difficult to move. If you have a boulder, you'll have massively high cholesterol due to the gene, and it will be very hard to budge with lifestyle or medication.

But you can also have polygenic high cholesterol, which means multiple genes are combining to raise your cholesterol. Each of those genes is like a large rock in the wheelbarrow. These large rocks can combine to weigh as much in the wheelbarrow as the boulder, but the individual rocks are much easier to unload.

A patient with a single dominant boulder gene almost always will need to be treated with medicine. Lifestyle choices can help them, but getting their cholesterol levels down almost always requires drugs. On the other hand, these less-dominant large-rock genes are much more responsive to lifestyle changes, allowing patients to lower their LDL cholesterol with diet and exercise.

In light of these genetic concerns, everyone should have a cholesterol test done in their teens or young adult years to determine if they have FH and begin treatment as soon as possible if they do. An early cholesterol test will also benefit those without FH who have high LDL because they can get their polygenic high cholesterol under control with lifestyle before they have a vascular catastrophe like a heart attack or stroke.

Curiously, if someone with FH lives past sixty-eight, their risk normalizes to that of the general population. Members of THINCS latch on to this to say, "See! Cholesterol can't be causing all these problems because even these people with genetic issues eventually have the same risk as everyone else."

This is an erroneous interpretation. In truth, it's not the

FH people sinking to the level of the general public but the general public catching up to those with the genetic problem. We have so much exposure to cholesterol throughout our lives now that our risk rises to the same level as those with FH.

That's not reassuring, is it?

Despite these genetic factors, high or low LDL cholesterol for most people is dictated by your lifestyle—what you eat, how much you eat, and how often you exercise. If you move from Tokyo to San Francisco, chances are high your LDL will go up as your diet adapts to the local cuisine. If you move from San Francisco to Tokyo, it will likely go down for the same reason.[88] We can take anyone, put them in a laboratory, change their diet, and regardless of genetics either raise or lower their LDL through diet. We can even predict the response accurately if we know their baseline cholesterol levels.

We've also examined populations whose LDL cholesterol has been under seventy their entire lives.[89] These people never develop atherosclerosis. These levels were common 150 years ago in the United States, but they are rare today.

The idea that cholesterol levels are driven entirely by genetics is impossible to sustain in the face of these facts. Most patients, regardless of their genes, can markedly improve high cholesterol numbers with big reductions in dietary saturated fat and dietary cholesterol. Genes can affect cholesterol, but genes are in the backseat of the car; lifestyle is driving the car. The people with the worst genes and the best lifestyle have no more risk than those with the best genes and worst lifestyle.[90]

There have been hundreds of epidemiological studies following people after their cholesterol has been measured. The depth of this research is staggering—200 different studies involving over 2 million participants with more than 20 million person-years of follow-up tracking more than 150,000 cardiovascular events.[91]

The results? The higher the LDL, the more likely people are to have heart disease. The lower the LDL, the less like they are to have heart disease. Medical science has very few associations that are this robust.

We also have many randomized controlled trials, which are considered the gold standard in medicine. These randomized trials clearly show that when we lower LDL cholesterol—with PCSK9 inhibitors, statins, cholestyramine, ezetimibe, or by bypassing the cholesterol absorption area of the small intestine with surgery—it reduces mortality from heart disease.

We should stop wasting money studying this issue. It's settled.

The higher your LDL cholesterol, the greater your chances are of a heart attack or stroke.

Modern humans on Western diets are the only organisms that have experimented with having widespread chronically elevated LDL, and the result is that atherosclerotic vascular disease is the number-one cause of death of human beings on Earth.

THE SIMPLE ANSWER

We know how to prevent cardiovascular disease and we know the cure for this most common cause of death in the world.

It's simple.

Everyone should spend as much of their lives with an LDL under seventy as possible. And people should start worrying about cholesterol much earlier in their life—in their teens and twenties—and figure out what lifestyle they need to adopt to get to that correct LDL cholesterol level and keep it there for the rest of their life. When you do that, you no longer have to worry about many of our most common health issues.

Yet we continue to contribute to this number-one cause of death with almost everything we eat. Our food system even allows teenagers and kids to develop LDL levels that are way too high.[92]

As adults, we continue with the habits that got us into trouble in the first place. People are unwilling to make the lifestyle choices—exercise and a diet low in saturated fat and cholesterol—that would make a difference, so as doctors we try to shock-absorb these horrifically high LDL levels with statin drugs and other medications. When we can't lower our LDL cholesterol because we're unwilling to change our diet, drugs become the only other option. Are we as healthcare providers okay with that?

Personally, it makes me uncomfortable.

The ads for statins always seem to suggest that diet and exercise "failed." But did they? Or did people just add broccoli, substitute chicken for beef, and skip ice cream once a week? In my experience, most people who take the guidelines seriously and really cut down on saturated fat can achieve LDL cholesterol levels under 70.

In the 1950s and 1960s, doctors frequently lowered cholesterol by putting people on a diet of rice and fruit, with total cholesterol dropping an average of 65 points. This shows how effective dietary changes can be in reducing cholesterol levels.[93]

The problem is that the people who are suffering from cardiovascular disease aren't fully aware of how much control they have over this condition. In many cases, people are confused about what to think. There is so much obfuscation and pushback from the food industry on products like coconut oil, beef, yogurt, and eggs that people have trouble making the connection.

We medical professionals have to take some responsibility for the chronically high LDL cholesterol problem in the US too.

Eric Rimm, a professor in the departments of epidemiology and nutrition at the Harvard T.H. Chan School of Public Health, has been involved in studies showing that a healthy, plant-based diet substantially lowers your risk of heart disease and type 2 diabetes.[94] He's the same researcher who attracted a hailstorm of scorn online for advising people to stop eating french fries or to at least limit their intake to six fries at any one meal.

But even Rimm was quoted as saying that we can't expect Americans to become vegetarian and give up all their dairy and eggs. He said it would be too extreme. Really? Well, what about the thousands of people each month who have to get bypasses and have their chests cut open? Isn't *that* too extreme? How about all the people who have to get angiograms or have stents put in their hearts? That seems like extreme treatment for a condition we know exactly how to prevent.

It seems much less extreme to suggest that people eat fruits, vegetables, beans, and grains as their primary sources of calories, as people have done through most of human history.

The more people understand that and demand that the food industry provide it, the fewer patients will develop cholesterol levels like the man who came to my office with a total cholesterol level over 1,100 mg/dL.

THE SOURCE OF LDL CHOLESTEROL

Nearly 400 different metabolic ward studies have examined LDL cholesterol. Metabolic ward studies are some of the most rigorous types of experiments researchers use. They are no fun. Patients are basically put in prison. If you're a subject in the study, you can't go in or out and no one can bring you anything. Everything you eat is carefully controlled and recorded.

When researchers in Great Britain did a meta-analysis of these 385 metabolic ward studies, they found that in study after study, the biggest driver of elevated LDL cholesterol was saturated fat.[95]

The results of these studies were used to create mathematical equations that accurately predict the change in cholesterol using changes in dietary saturated fat and cholesterol (see sidebar). These equations have been verified by multiple researchers in multiple countries in both laboratory and free-living scenarios.[96]

KEYS EQUATION: CHANGE IN SERUM CHOLESTEROL CONCENTRATION

$$(MMOL/L) = 0.031(2DSF - DPUF) + 1.5\sqrt{DCH}$$

The Keys equation predicts how saturated and polyunsaturated fatty acids influence serum cholesterol levels. The equation is based on Ancel Keys' findings that saturated fats increase total and LDL cholesterol at twice the rate that polyunsaturated fats decrease those cholesterol levels.

Here's how to interpret the equation: Dsf is the change in percentage of dietary energy from saturated fats, Dpuf is the change in percentage of dietary energy from polyunsaturated fats, and Dch is the change in intake of dietary cholesterol. This equation is often used by dietitians when developing low-fat diets for patients.

Here's why the Keys equation is important: it allows us to predict with good accuracy what direction and how much cholesterol levels will increase when your saturated fat consumption goes up.

This equation is a half-century old, and during those fifty years no one has tried to disprove it. Most articles attacking cholesterol don't bring up the equation.

That's because Keys' equation, like the laws of gravity, accurately predicts the future: if we know your baseline cholesterol, we can predict with accuracy what your cholesterol will be if you increase your saturated fat intake. When you increase saturated fat, your cholesterol goes up. When you decrease saturated fat and increase polyunsaturated fat, cholesterol goes down. The equation shows this and no one has ever suggested the equation isn't accurate.

It is absolutely solid, undisputed science that high LDL cholesterol causes heart disease and that heart disease is the number-one cause of death in the world. And these equations show just as decisively that high dietary saturated fat uniformly and linearly leads to high LDL cholesterol.

This connection is so well established that it's embarrassing to suggest that the science is flawed in any way. A diet rich in saturated fat increases LDL cholesterol. High LDL cholesterol causes heart disease. Heart disease kills more people each year than any other cause of death.

Yet, you still have a group of people who for some reason or another are trying to push back against the idea that saturated fat is problematic. To disprove the connection between high LDL and dietary saturated fat, you would have to conduct your own metabolic ward trials. You would have to feed your patients animal fats, tropical oils, and/or dairy products rich in saturated fat and show that the diet did not elevate LDL cholesterol. But no one is doing that. They aren't doing that because they know what the results would be. (Hint: the results would not show saturated fat is good for you.)

That's why there isn't a single medical organization in the world that has suggested LDL cholesterol is not a concern. There isn't a single dietary guideline in the world that recommends you should not worry about saturated fat. There isn't a single group of dietitians, cardiologists, or atherosclerosis researchers that has suggested anything other than standard guideline advice: you should keep your saturated fat intake below 10 percent of your total calories, or 6 percent or less if you're trying to reverse disease. What's more, there isn't a single medical or science group that recommends people increase the amount of saturated fat in their diet.

So when you read about people losing weight and "feeling great" on low-carb, high-fat ketogenic diets, take the news with a few grains of salt. You may lose some weight by cutting your carbs to 30 grams a day and consuming as much butter, cheese, and milk as you like, but you certainly aren't doing your cardiovascular system any favors and you are setting yourself up for a whole range of problems—from heart attack to diabetes to cancer to strokes—in the future. When these trimmed-down ketogenic devotees keel over in five or ten years from cardiovascular disease, no one will mention how great they look.

ADOPTING A BETTER DIET OURSELVES

As healers, it's vital that we start eating better ourselves. It's not difficult to find an orthopedist, primary care doctor, physical therapist, or nurse who has diabetes, suffers from obesity, or has a fatty liver like I had. Many of us aren't willing to cut down our saturated fat because we see it as a big limitation in our lives. I felt that way before I finally took steps to change how I ate. I never doubted that this stuff was bad for me, but I would still buy a block of cheddar cheese at the supermarket and eat it throughout the week. I knew it was something I shouldn't be eating, but it still took me a long time to eliminate it from my diet.

Similarly, when I'm talking to healthcare pros, they don't dispute the importance of LDL cholesterol and they don't push back on saturated fat. They know saturated fat is bad for them, but they don't take it seriously enough to reduce their consumption of the foods that contain so much of it.

"I know it's bad for me, but I really like my bacon and eggs for breakfast," they'll say.

Our country's attitude about saturated fat today is comparable to what it was with smoking back in the fifties. Back then, the problem everyone talked about was *excessive* smoking, not smoking in general. The answer for the guy smoking two packs of Marlboros every day was to cut down to one pack and switch to Chesterfields. Doctors who advised against smoking at all were labeled "anti-tobacco activists."

Then a younger generation of doctors came along and learned the full scope of the problems caused by smoking. The 1964 US Surgeon General's report (published a year before I was born) on smoking and health linked smoking to lung cancer and heart disease. That made it much harder for those who still smoked to defend the habit or to continue to not advise their patients to stop smoking. Not being able to defend it, most doctors quit, and today smoking is rare among physicians. Less than 1 percent of all doctors smoke. What's more, smoking is not controversial anymore, and there is a consensus among healthcare professionals to restrict it in any way we can.

Unfortunately, we don't have a report on saturated fat that's comparable to the 1964 Surgeon General's report on smoking. That might have something to do with the fact that the USDA doesn't want to come out and say meat, fish, dairy, eggs, and tropical oils are all toxic and should be dramatically limited compared to current practice. The USDA has historically supported and promoted many of those products, so it would be hard for them to make that pirouette.

Still, you could argue that the threat from saturated fat is just as serious as tobacco smoking once was. At its height of popularity, about half the population smoked cigarettes. But 98.5 percent of people fail to meet the standards for a healthy diet.[97]

Healthcare systems aren't taking this issue seriously enough. Patients aren't taking this seriously enough, either. We live in a media and market landscape that doesn't support significant changes in our food habits because so much profit is at stake.

To give you an idea, Cargill, a major meat supplier, has annual revenues of $137 billion.[98] Tyson Foods sells over $40 billion annually.[99] With this level of revenue at stake, why wouldn't a company take aggressive steps to control the media narrative about their product? When healthcare professionals and researchers recommend that we all reduce our consumption of these products by 90 percent, wouldn't you expect those companies to fight back? With that level of revenue at stake, it's worth spending billions to control the narrative. It's just reasonable business.

As a result of this controlled media narrative, we don't appreciate how easy it is to avoid cardiovascular disease and all the other maladies that come from high serum cholesterol and a diet too heavy in saturated fat.

Today, the lean man who came into our office with an LDL cholesterol reading of 1,100 is keeping his cholesterol numbers low by eating a largely plant-based diet. He still occasionally eats foods higher in saturated fat, but that's only because his wife insists on it and he wants his wife to be happy. He says the only time he suffers chest pains at all now is when he argues with his wife.

Chapter 5

DIABETES: FAT IS WORSE THAN SUGAR

When I was a medical resident on a surgical rotation, we performed operations on some young people who were lean and healthy and on other patients with obesity. When we opened the abdomen of the lean patients, you could clearly see their internal organs—their intestines, liver, pancreas, spleen, and some spider-webby-looking material called omentum.

When we opened the abdominal wall of the other patients, however, the most dominant feature was the yellow globules of fat attached to the organs and omentum. This intra-abdominal visceral fat is called appendices epiploicae, and sometimes you could barely make out the outline of the internal organs beneath it. You didn't need a lot of complicated blood tests to conclude that these obese patients probably had diabetes.

In the medical field, people with diabetes are not hard to find.

The latest report from the Centers for Disease Control and Prevention found that more than 100 million Americans are living with either diabetes or prediabetes, a condition that frequently leads to type 2 diabetes within five years if it's not addressed. One in ten people in the United States have full-blown diabetes, and 1.5 million new cases are diagnosed each year. One in four people with diabetes don't even know they have it.

Diabetes is increasing around the world as more developing countries transition to the high-fat, highly processed diet of an industrialized culture. In China, where diabetes was once rare, the disease spread so rapidly in the last thirty years that China now has the worst epidemic on the planet.[100]

And let's not kid ourselves and think that diabetes is merely an annoyance. It's a serious disease. It makes you as likely to die from a heart attack as someone who's already had a heart attack. It makes you as likely to have a stroke as someone who has already had a stroke. It's the number-one cause of blindness in our country. It's the number-one cause of amputations. It's associated with a massively higher likelihood of erectile dysfunction. It's even associated with developing cancer of the colon.[101]

People with diabetes spend a lot of money getting treatment. Americans with diabetes spend more than $16 billion a year on dialysis, and they also spend money on doctors' visits to get their blood tested and their eyes examined. They take medication—shots, pills, or a combination of the two. One of my patients was spending over $450 per month on his diabetes supplies and medications. That's enough to pay the lease on a Mercedes!

If someone with diabetes dies of a heart attack, we say they died of a heart attack. But did they die of the heart attack alone or did they die of their diabetes? Usually, it's a combination of the two.

Diabetes is a horrific disease, and despite its prevalence and spread, we in healthcare still seem confused about what to tell our patients who either have the disease or have prediabetes and are likely to get it. We all prescribe more exercise for our patients with diabetes and we also urge our patients to lose weight. Some of us give our patients the biguanide drug Metformin to help delay or prevent type 2 diabetes.

But how many of us are warning our patients to eliminate or avoid saturated fat—one of the deadliest causes of diabetes around the globe?

Certainly, not enough.

THE MECHANISM

Type 2 diabetes is a semi-adaptive response to absorbing more calories than you burn. Since your body is naturally a hoarder—an evolutionary adaption to primitive times when we didn't know where our next meal was coming from—most excess calories are stored as fat. The standard treatment for diabetes is to prescribe Metformin, but controlling diet and exercise is a simpler solution. If you can get patients to eat less and burn more calories than they consume, they will lose weight and their diabetes will get better.

A group of researchers in the United Kingdom did exactly this in a study where they put a group of diabetes patients on an intensive weight management program. The patients had body-mass indexes of between 27 and 45 kg/m^2, and part of the group was put on a carefully restricted diet of 825 to 853 calories a day. Eighty-six percent of the patients who lost 15 kilograms (33 pounds) or more were in remission[102] and patients who lost weight reported that their quality of life increased. They were able to resume normal physiological meal tolerances, including eating *carbohydrates*, after their weight loss.

Most people in the healthcare field aren't doing enough to convince people with diabetes to focus more carefully on their consumption of saturated fat, though, which is uniquely bad and uniquely likely to cause the physiological changes that lead to diabetes.

When you compare patients whose diets are nearly identical—the percent of their calories from fat is the same, the levels of protein, carbohydrate, and total calories are the same—the patients who have the highest percentage of their calories from saturated fat have the greatest level of insulin resistance. We'll talk about why this is in the next chapter, but for now it's important to know that when the percentage of calories from saturated fat goes up, so does a patient's insulin resistance. And insulin resistance is the primary physiological change associated with the development of type 2 diabetes.

Saturated fat isn't the sole cause of diabetes; it's just one of the more reliable and powerful causes.

The first change on the road leading to diabetes is the development of fatty liver.[103] Researchers in Finland studied several dozen overweight patients and found that those who consumed more saturated fat had 55 percent more fat build-up in the liver than those who overconsumed unsaturated fat or sugar.[104] The correlation between high-sugar diets and high saturated fat diets is incredibly strong; if you're eating a lot of sugar, you are almost certainly eating a lot of saturated fat as well, as many sugary foods, such as brownies and milkshakes, are also high in saturated fat. But people instinctively want to believe that diabetes is caused by sugar consumption. They see people who eat loads of sugar get diabetes and they think, *Oh it must be the sugar.*

The evidence does not support that.

Anyone who really digs into the science of insulin resistance finds that saturated fat is the primary cause of the disease. In fact, the physiology of fatty liver and the physiology of diabetes are indistinguishable—and both are caused by the buildup of the visceral intracellular fat inside the abdominal cavity that I witnessed so often during my surgical rotation.

HOW SATURATED FAT CAUSES DIABETES

To help you explain this to your patients, let's look at how type 2 diabetes develops and the role fat plays in that development.

Type 2 diabetes is largely a disease of calorie excess.

When researchers want to study type 2 diabetes in rodents, they feed them diets high in total fat. This reliably gives mice and rats diabetes that we can reverse by changing the food.[105] This isn't the only possible way to do it; it's just the easiest. If you can get the rodents to overeat any kind of food, especially the common Western diet many people eat, you can predictably produce diabetes because the disease develops when you can't store any more of your food for energy.

The protein and starches we eat are converted into glucose, or sugar, before they can be used as the body's preferred fuel. Insulin, a hormone produced by the pancreas, helps glucose move into tissues that are low in glucose and allows them to store it for use as glycogen. Insulin works to facilitate movement of glucose into energy-hungry cells like a thermostat works on temperature. When a cell has low glucose, insulin helps that cell take up more of it. When a cell's glycogen stores are full, insulin sensitivity is dialed down.

Continuing the thermometer metaphor, insulin resistance (IR) occurs when the temperature outside a room gets too high for the air conditioning to keep up. This is the telltale sign of both prediabetes and type 2 diabetes, and it's triggered when stored fat builds up in our liver, muscles, and pancreas, creating toxic fatty acids and free radicals.

The easiest way to get IR, however, is a high-fat meal. IR can occur just three hours after the consumption of too much saturated fat and persists for up to twelve hours after it starts.[106]

A healthy liver's job is to produce blood sugar for our brain between meals. When we eat, the insulin shuts down that liver glucose production. But when that insulin no longer works on the insulin-resistant liver, the liver continues pumping out more sugar after we've eaten. Just as a room will heat up when the air conditioner can't keep up because too much heat is coming in, the blood sugar starts to rise when the insulin can't work properly to turn off sugar production in the liver. This, in turn, prompts the pancreas to produce more insulin, which increases the amount of fat deposited in the liver, leading to a feed-forward loop of ever higher sugars, liver fats, and insulin levels.

It isn't fun.

This continues to get worse until the kidneys start peeing out enough sugar to cause net weight loss. But at this point the person with diabetes is miserable; their mouth is dry, they're running to the bathroom all the time, and they can't stop their ravenous hunger. We call it polyuria, polydipsia, and polyphagia, and these are the primary symptoms people present when they get a diagnosis of diabetes.

The fatty liver directs excess fat back into the blood-stream, where it travels to the pancreas and kills the pancreatic beta cells that produce insulin. Researchers have grown pancreatic beta cells in culture and found out that palmitic acid, the most common saturated fat in food, actually causes beta cells to commit suicide in a process called apoptosis.[107]

Now you're in a real fix; you are insulin resistant. Reduced insulin production in your fatty pancreas and fat blocking the liver from responding to the insulin you have are prompting your blood sugar to skyrocket. This is going to drive up the room temperature and cause dangerously high heat.

This is type 2 diabetes.

FATS CAUSE INSULIN RESISTANCE; SATURATED FAT CAUSES EVEN MORE

Saturated fat has the short-term effect of killing pancreatic beta cells (something we'll discuss in greater detail in the next chapter) as well as the long-term effect on your muscles, liver, and pancreas. Saturated fatty acids, such as palmitic acid from palm oil, (where it gets its name), meat, dairy, and eggs, contribute to insulin resistance.

Most cases of diabetes are people with type 2 diabetes,

or adult-onset diabetes. This accounts for 90 to 95 percent of all cases of diabetes. Type 1 diabetes occurs when people are unable to make insulin and usually appears during childhood or adolescence. Type 2 diabetes, primarily brought on by low-quality diet and a sedentary lifestyle, is more common in people older than forty. All other causes are quite rare, and I won't address those in this book.

While the incidence of type 2 diabetes is strongly associated with the proportion of saturated fat in our blood, the fat is not the only factor. Most diets high in saturated fat are animal-based diets rich in total fat, trans fat, cholesterol, protein, heme iron, and phosphatidylcholine, all of which have been scientifically implicated in cardiovascular disease, cancer, and diabetes. You can't just eliminate the saturated fat and expect diabetes to go away. It helps to eat a plant-based diet rich in nutrients, fiber, and whole grains, but if you merely douse your healthy dish with oils—especially tropical oils high in saturated fat—you aren't helping yourself any.

Going back nearly one hundred years to the 1930s, researchers have repeatedly shown that a diet based on vegetables, fruits, grains, and beans is an effective treatment for diabetes. Those who eat meat one or more times a week have significantly higher rates of diabetes while those who stick with a plant-based diet are nearly 80 percent less likely to get diabetes.[108]

Researchers at the Imperial College of London who compared omnivores to vegans, all of whom had comparable body mass indexes, body fat percentages, activity levels, and caloric intake, found that the plant-eaters had better insulin sensitivity, blood sugar, insulin levels, and pancreatic beta-cell function than their meat-eating counterparts.[109] In 1979, a group of men with diabetes were put on a high carbohydrate, high-fiber diet, and in just over two weeks, half of the men were able to stop taking insulin altogether.[110]

If your patients think merely cutting back on meat will help them, kindly suggest they think again. These patients may need to drastically cut back their meat consumption. In a 2014 study of more than 4,000 Taiwanese Buddhists, the men who were strictly vegetarian had 50 percent fewer cases of diabetes than those who ate meat. Vegetarian women had 75 percent fewer cases. And those eating meat were consuming what most Americans would consider tiny portions; the Taiwanese men ate just 8 percent of the amount of meat an average American male consumes and the women ate less than 3 percent of the meat an average American woman eats. So even small portions cause problems.[111]

Other studies[112] suggest that the source of dietary fat also plays a part in increasing the risk for type 2 diabetes. When researchers at Harvard teamed up with colleagues from Universitat Rovira i Virgili in Spain to track 3,349 Spanish adults for about four and a half years, they found that people who consumed larger amounts of saturated fats and animal fats got twice as many cases of diabetes as those who consumed a smaller amount. Butter and cheese contributed greatly to an increased risk of diabetes. Sometimes the effect of a high-fat meal on your body's blood-sugar-and-insulin system is head-snappingly fast. In one case, a group of healthy men in Germany consumed a drink of palm oil that contained as much saturated fat as a cheeseburger and order of fries. Their insulin sensitivity declined and researchers noted an increase in fat deposits in the liver *that day*. Their metabolism became similar to those with diabetes.[113]

IT'S NOT ALL CARB RESTRICTION

As we mentioned before, the biggest misperception healthcare providers and patients have about diabetes is that it's caused by the overconsumption of sugar. To complicate matters further, we now have a lot of unscientific, low-carb bloggers, journalists, and nonspecialist doctors declaring that carbs are causing diabetes and that we have to severely limit them from our diet. These same low-carb proponents also endorse high-fat ketogenic and Atkins-style diets.

In the face of this misguided advice and the alarming numbers of people with type 2 diabetes, those of us in healthcare need to understand that saturated fat is a primary cause of diabetes. Our patients need to know this too.

They need to know that people who eat the most whole grains have fewer cases of diabetes. They need to know that people who eat unprocessed, unrefined starchy carbohydrates have fewer cases of diabetes. They should also know that experts have recommended diets based on vegetables, fruits, grains, and beans for people with diabetes since the 1930s.

Here's a simple experiment that underscores the wisdom of a plant-based diet for people with diabetes. In 1927, a Texas physician named Shirley Sweeney ran his medical students through four different two-day regimens.[114] In the first regimen, the group ate mainly carbohydrates in the form of syrup, cotton candy, and starches. In the second regimen the group ate primarily protein. The third phase was eating nothing but fats and in the fourth phase, the students ate nothing.

On the third day of each phase, all the students drank a

beverage with a set amount of glucose in it and had their blood sugar monitored.

After their carbohydrate diet, the group showed stable blood sugar levels. But blood sugar levels shot up after the other three other regimens. The high-fat diet triggered the worst results; sugar levels in the students after that regimen were similar to patients with severe diabetes. These results were replicated by others, and ten years later, people with diabetes put on a low-fat diet based on rice, fruit, and fruit juice saw big improvements[115] in their condition. Even patients with type 1 diabetes were able to reduce their insulin doses and enjoyed improved vision when they ate this way.

One of the most prominent specialists in diabetes was Elliot P. Joslin, whose name is associated with the famous Joslin Diabetes Clinics. He had this nailed back in 1930 as well:

> I believe the chief cause of premature atherosclerosis in diabetes, save for advancing age, is an excess of fat, an excess of fat in the body (obesity), an excess of fat in the diet, and an excess of fat in the blood. With an excess of fat, diabetes begins and from an excess of fat (people with diabetes) die, formerly of coma, recently of atherosclerosis.[116]

This statement forecast perfectly the modern experience

of the nation of China. The Chinese have dropped their consumption of rice dramatically and increased their protein and fat consumption. Their rate of diabetes is one of the highest in the world. Where once just 1 percent of the Chinese had diabetes, now close to 10 percent of its population has the disease. The percentage of overweight people in China has also gone up as a result of these dietary changes.[117]

Despite these results from China, many doctors continue to advise their patients with diabetes to avoid eating all carbs, instead of just restricting sugars. It's time we stopped giving that advice.

We test for diabetes with the hemoglobin A1c test, which tells you the patient's average blood sugar level over the past two to three months. The normal range for this test is 4 to 5.6 percent, and hemoglobin A1c levels between 5.7 and 6.4 mean you have prediabetes. A level over 6.4 means you have diabetes. Hemoglobin A1c levels are determined by two measurements taken at least two months apart.

I've had patients with hemoglobin A1cs of 13.6 percent, which is very high and means they have diabetes. But when they follow a very low-fat, high-carbohydrate diet with a lot of starchy carbs but not a lot of sugar, we can normalize their blood sugar levels within three or four months.

If you learn anything from this book, I hope you learn that although sugar is bad, it is not the cause of diabetes. Fat—particularly saturated fat—is the primary culprit, especially when someone eats too many calories.[118] Sugar is bad because when it is eaten in excess, the body turns excess sugar beyond what's needed for energy and storage into saturated fat (primarily palmitic acid), which causes insulin resistance and high cholesterol and gout and all the other bad things associated with sugar.

Study after study in laboratory animals, cell culture studies, and observations of human beings suggests that it's not carbohydrates causing diabetes but saturated fat.[119] It's basic chemistry and physiology. Of course you can make the picture more confusing by causing massive weight loss (see box). If low-carb proponents want to prove that carbohydrates cause diabetes, they should at least conduct laboratory studies or metabolic ward studies showing high-fat diets improve insulin sensitivity.

But we don't see that.

We don't see people feeding people with diabetes loads of saturated fat and measuring improvement in their insulin resistance. In most low-carb trials, researchers don't even run glucose tolerance tests at the end of the study. They perhaps skip that step because they know the results will disprove their thesis.

START-UP SELLS QUESTIONABLE
DIABETES TREATMENT

In the last few years, a Bay Area startup has burst on the diabetes scene with a dietary plan it says can reverse type 2 diabetes.

Virta Health charges people $400 a month for online counseling and medical oversight to help patients manage their diabetes. The company gives members a health coach, a physician, and peer support and puts members on a low-carb, fat-rich ketogenic diet that limits carbs to 30 grams a day but doesn't put any restrictions on how much you eat or how much fat you consume.

If you believe the company's published research, you'd think they were on to something. In 2018, its one-year, peer-reviewed results[120] showed that 60 percent of the patients who completed the Virta program were able to control their diabetes and 94 percent were able to reduce or eliminate their insulin use. Patients lost an average of 7 percent of their body weight.[121]

The efficacy of the program was touted through a 2017 study published in the Journal of Medical Internet Research, a new digital-only medical journal. A year later, Virta published a second peer-reviewed paper in *Cardiovascular Diabetology*,[122] claiming that their treatment program "showed significant improvement in 22 of 26 markers of cardiovascular disease risk in patients with type 2 diabetes."

Before you send all your patients with diabetes to sign up with Virta, which has attracted $45 million in venture capital funding, you might want to point out a few problems with its findings[123]:

- Every author involved in the 2017 Virta study disclosed they had a financial stake in the company.[124] They were highly motivated to make the program appear to be miraculously effective.
- Several authors disclosed they received funding from Atkins Nutritionals, the National Dairy Council, and the Palm Oil Board. These are all purveyors of products and food rich in saturated fat.
- The study only included patients who signed up with Virta. It was neither an observational trial nor a randomized trial. There was no genuine control group, and 10 percent of the 262 adults involved in the study dropped out—a significant number.
- The comparator group for the study was a group of people who wanted to sign up for the counseling offered by Virta but ultimately chose not to hire Virta for $400 a month. This, by itself, makes the results of Virta's "scientific" study utterly predictable; it's obvious that anyone paying $400 a month to manage their

diabetes by a doctor is going to have better outcomes than someone going it alone.

- Virta claims it got people off their diabetes medicine, but the number of patients on Metformin actually increased, as did the number of patients taking GLP-1 inhibitors, which are potent weight-loss drugs.
- The study claims there were no bad outcomes from the program even though they report that two patients died in the course of the research.

While it may be true that some people lose weight on ketogenic diets, the Virta research does little to counterbalance the many studies—conducted by doctors who don't have a financial stake in the outcome[125] and who follow far more patients over a significantly longer period of time[126]—that show that low-carb, high-fat diets are associated with a higher risk of all-cause and cardiovascular mortality. Although Virta touts its own research, including a recent study in the journal *Diabetes Therapy*,[127] it fails to mention these studies on its website.

Virta is not a reliable study in any way. It is an investor precis.

ADVICE FOR HEALTHCARE PROVIDERS

I don't want you to get the idea that keeping your patients away from saturated fat will prevent them from getting diabetes. That's not the case. You can avoid all saturated fat and instead eat loads of polyunsaturated fat and carbohydrates in excess and still develop diabetes. You still need to advise your patients with diabetes to lose weight and get more exercise.

But your patients need to understand the unique and deadly power that saturated fat can have to raise insulin resistance, cause fatty liver disease, and trigger diabetes. One 2017 study in *The American Journal of Clinical Nutrition* found that people who consume higher amounts of saturated fat and animal fats are twice as likely to develop diabetes as those who consume less.[128]

Most people don't want to hear that they have to give up meat entirely. But as healthcare providers, we have a responsibility to warn our patients about the risks of eating meat. Most people didn't want to hear about the dangers of cigarette smoking either, but the healthcare system didn't care and told all patients the truth about cigarettes and smoking.

When it comes to meat, the simple truth is that even small amounts can be damaging.

We don't know exactly what it is, but we have good reasons to think it's probably a combination of saturated fat, inflammatory responses, heme iron, dangerous byproducts of the cooking process, and other components found in meat.

A 2013 study that followed 17,000 people for nearly twelve years found an 8 percent increase in the diabetes risk for every fifty grams of meat consumed each day. Just fifty grams.[129] A single chicken breast with the bone and skin removed is about 170 grams!

Patients, if you're reading this, you need to understand that to reduce your diabetes risk, you must reduce your saturated fat intake, and since saturated fats are primarily found in animal-based foods, you have to decide if those foods should be part of your regular menu. But even vegans who eat no animal products at all can still get all the harms from a diet rich in saturated fat if they indulge in fake meats, cheeses, snacks, and desserts made with coconut or palm oil—since they are also loaded with saturated fat.

While the risks of developing diabetes might be compelling enough for patients to reduce their saturated fat, there are other dangers to worry about. One of them is a relatively new culprit that we're just starting to hear about: ceramide. Read on to find out how this waxy material once thought to be innocuous is raising new red flags for people who eat diets high in saturated fat.

Chapter 6

CERAMIDE

While diabetes is often associated with obesity, doctors have known for years that slender people can also develop the disease and that some people with obesity are unexpectedly healthy. They just didn't know why.

In recent years, however, an explanation has emerged: ceramide.

Ceramide, like cholesterol, is a lipid made of big, waxy molecules. It is similar in structure and characteristics to ear wax. In fact, the chemical name for ear wax, cerumen, comes from the same root word as ceramide. Both ceramide and cholesterol are sticky, greasy molecules that are used in small quantities to hold cell membranes together.

But their similarities don't end there. Ceramide, like cholesterol, is a product of a diet high in saturated fat and it plays a role in diabetes, heart disease, hypertension, body-wide inflammation, cancer, and, as we'll talk more about in a future chapter, dementia. When you are consuming high levels of saturated fat, you are making way too much ceramide in the pancreas, liver, heart, and brain.

Before 2000, no one really thought much about ceramide. If you told someone in medical school that you were going to study ceramide, they'd look at you quizzically and ask why you cared about ear wax. Today, thanks to better scientific methods for detecting it, we know that ceramide is a significant player in all the chronic metabolic diseases of civilization.

SHOULD YOU BE VEGAN?

Small amounts of animals products have negative effects, but a diet that includes only small amounts of animal products will be infinitely better than a diet that includes large amounts.

And vegan diets can be just as dangerous if loaded with saturated fat. In fact, you can design a diet that includes some animal product that is much healthier than a high-saturated-fat vegan diet. But the healthiest diets will never be high in animal products.

The choice to be fully vegan, inclusive of cosmetics, clothing, and food, fits in very well with the diet that I find most beneficial for health. There is not one single reason I adopted veganism, but I definitely had an easier time than many people will, since I had been vegetarian from birth.

The factors that led to my decision to be vegan were a combination of improved health, ethics, and environmental stewardship. At least 70 percent of the grain produced in the United States is fed to livestock,[130] and the world's 1.3 billion cattle occupy nearly a quarter of the Earth's land, including vast tracks of tropical forests that have been cleared (often by fire) to create pastures for cows.[131] Why do we commit so much of our precious resources for animal products that cause so many public health problems?

If you choose to be vegan, you should make sure you take a vitamin B12 supplement and be tested for other vitamins, including vitamin D. Many people who are not vegan are still deficient, so people eating a plant-based diet should have these levels checked regularly.

Some people tell me they must have animal protein or they feel horrible. That may be true, but I can't tell because I can't get inside their body and feel what they feel. It's possible it's all psychological and it's possible it's based on some real physiological change.

What we do know is that no one has ever been hospitalized because of an animal protein deficiency—and that plant proteins contain all the amino acids necessary for people to thrive. From a physiological standpoint, you don't need animal products.

However, if you feel you must have animal protein, then there is one source that is by far the best, and it's not the one you think.

I'm talking about pulverized insects.

Any objective analysis shows that pulverized insects, such as cricket flour, are the most ecologically sensitive and healthy animal protein available to us. It's high in protein and has almost no saturated fat. If you aren't craving it, it's almost certainly because of your own psychology. Throughout evolution, primates have only ever been herbivores or insectivores, so insects may be easier to get used to than you first thought. According to the Food and Agriculture Organization of the United Nations, 25 percent of the world's population eats bugs regularly,[132] and the USDA reports that Americans inadvertently eat 1–2 pounds of pulverized insects annually.

THE CERAMIDE PROBLEM

Many people know that overeating produces excess fatty

acids that are typically stored in the body as triglycerides or burned for energy. But according to a University of Utah College of Health study from 2016,[133] those fatty acids can produce excess ceramide in some people. When that happens, the ceramide restricts how the body burns calories and how it responds to insulin. The buildup of ceramide may also cause adipose tissue to stop working correctly, allowing fat to spill out into the body and pose danger to peripheral tissues, the heart, and blood vessels.

The three-year study at Utah found that mice given excess ceramide became unresponsive to insulin and had an increased risk of getting diabetes and fatty liver disease. Adding excess ceramide to human fat cells produced the same effect. The researchers say the findings could explain why some skinny people will get diabetes or fatty liver disease: some people are predisposed to turning excess dietary fat into toxic ceramide.[134]

The Utah study builds on research that goes back twenty years in which scientists would drip saturated and unsaturated fatty acids on the beta cells of the pancreas. Beta cells are found within clusters of cells called islets and make insulin that controls glucose levels in the blood. You can be insulin resistant and not have glucose problems as long as your beta cells are healthy. People with type 1 diabetes get the disease because their body mistakenly destroys those beta cells.

Those older studies found that the damage caused to beta cells by saturated fatty acids was much worse than the damage caused by unsaturated fatty acids; ceramide that built up from saturated fatty acid actually caused the beta cells to kill themselves, a process called apoptosis.[135] That, of course, is not good. As diabetic physiology progresses, the more insulin resistant you are, the more insulin your pancreas needs to produce to keep up. You need those beta cells.

After researchers had established that saturated fat and the ceramide it produced were bad for your beta cells, other scientists went on to show the exact receptors on which ceramide works, how it blocks the mechanism of insulin, how ceramide damages the endoplasmic reticulum and mitochondria in the pancreas, and how it blocks the insulin receptor in the liver.

HEALTH PROBLEMS ASSOCIATED WITH CERAMIDE

If you needed yet another reason to advise patients to reduce the amount of saturated fat in their diet, ceramide might do the trick. It seems like every year brings a new flurry of scientific findings about the dangers of elevated ceramide levels.

Our bodies need a certain amount of ceramide. Ceramide accounts for about half of the fat in our skin and helps impede infectious agents while preventing water loss. It's often touted as a safe skin treatment. At the right level, ceramide also helps form cellular membranes and, according to researchers at the Sanford Burnham Prebys Medical Discovery Institute, helps ensure a strong cardiac function.

But too much ceramide wreaks havoc. The Sanford Burnham Prebys researchers, for instance, found that elevated ceramides play a significant role in lipotoxic cardiomyopathy, a heart condition that often afflicts people with diabetes and the obese. They also found that ceramide can affect specific protein molecules in a way that leads to cell death and heart muscle problems. Researchers there are now studying how ceramides affect breast cancer in patients with obesity.[136]

Unfortunately, the problems related to elevated ceramide levels don't end there. Researchers at Baylor College of Medicine found that ceramide is a key player in the development of a form of Parkinson's disease,[137] and another study showed ceramide plays a role in the development of multiple sclerosis. This may partially explain the success of patients following Dr. Roy Swank's diet for this condition, which is specifically designed to be very low in saturated fat.[138] Building on that finding, a report in the journal *Clinical Science* found that ceramide increases white blood cell infiltration into the central nervous system, resulting in inflammation in patients with MS.[139]

Ceramide also seems to reduce the metabolic activity of fat tissue. When the researchers in Utah blocked ceramide synthesis in human cells, they found fat cells burned more calories and became more sensitive to insulin. Reducing elevated ceramide increased the amount of a body's beige or brown fat, which is known as the "good fat" because it's full of iron-rich mitochondria that burn energy instead of merely packing it away.[134] Researchers say figuring out how to convert white fat to brown fat would help in treating diabetes and obesity, and learning how to manage ceramide is now part of that effort.

CERAMIDE AND CHOLESTEROL

There are apparent similarities between ceramide and cholesterol. Both are needed in small quantities for cellular membranes, both are complex pathways that produce many different lipids, and both are markers and potential causes of cardiovascular disease.

Both also have a relationship with cancer. Cancer cells tend to have higher concentrations of cholesterol and ceramide, but the jury is still out on whether the cholesterol or ceramide cause cancer or just feed it. One study looked at malignant tumor tissue samples from breast cancer patients and found significantly elevated amounts of ceramide when compared to normal tissue samples from the same people, showing that the breast cancer cells were preferentially taking up or making large amounts of it.[140]

The association between ceramide and diabetes in humans is particularly strong. A study in the *Journal of Pediatric Endocrinology and Metabolism* found that in female children and adolescents with type 2 diabetes, ceramide levels are elevated.[141] Another study from the Cleveland Clinic found that patients with type 2 diabetes had much higher concentrations of total ceramide, and that insulin sensitivity was inversely correlated with total ceramide.[142] In other words, as total ceramide goes up, the more resistant you are to insulin.

While there is still a lot of research to be done on ceramide, what we know now is enough to sound the alarm. The research is devastatingly strong. Yet perhaps one-eighth of 1 percent of the population has even heard of ceramide and even less are aware that it's dangerous. How can that be? The only explanation is that the media are not interested in studies that show saturated fat is bad for you and they are very interested in studies that suggest the opposite.

Even the dairy industry, which as we've noted earlier in the book has helped manipulate the science to suggest that people don't have to worry about saturated fat in milk, cheese, and butter, is aware of the dangers posed by ceramide to their own cows.

In one study, researchers gave cows triglycerides—which are composed primarily of saturated fat—through an IV. The goal of the study was to help determine the best diet for producing the most milk. But this infusion of saturated fat promoted ceramide accumulation and fatty liver in the cows.[143] In another study, researchers found they should be giving cows polyunsaturated fatty acids instead of saturated fatty acids.[144]

The irony here is that the dairy industry is happy to sell people products that are rich in saturated fat but they won't feed saturated fat to their own cows because it makes them desperately sick.

CERAMIDE AND CARDIOVASCULAR DISEASE

Not only does ceramide act in the pancreas to cause diabetes and in the liver to cause insulin resistance, it also can cause damage to the heart by causing ventricular thickening, weakened contractility, and heart failure.[145]

When researchers put palmitate onto human cardiac cells that have been grown in culture, ceramide develops and causes insulin resistance, oxidative stress, and destruction of the mitochondria, effectively causing these heart cells to kill themselves. This is not the result you want for someone who might already be experiencing reduced blood flow to their heart caused by cholesterol and narrowed arteries.

In fact, researchers at the Mayo Clinic found that ceramide can predict who will have a heart attack, stroke, or heart surgery.[146] Even when a person has no blocked arteries and a low level of LDL cholesterol, high levels of ceramide increase the risk of a cardiac event by three or four times.

The oversupply of fat to tissues that aren't designed to store it leads to diabetes and cardiovascular disease, but the oversupply of a sphingolipid such as ceramide is particularly hard on your body. Too much ceramide disrupts insulin sensitivity, kills pancreatic beta cells, and affects your arteries' ability to expand and contract to control blood flow. When researchers in Utah were able to inhibit ceramide biosynthesis in rodents, they saw improvements in the animals' diabetes, cardiomyopathy, insulin resistance, atherosclerosis, and steatohepatitis.[147]

When you look at all the ceramide studies, most of which have been done in the last ten years, they all point in the same direction: you should not be eating a diet high in saturated fats. When you look at the meal plans for some of the low-carb, high-fat diets that are out there, up to 85 percent of the calories are coming from fat and 50 percent of those fats are coming from saturated fat. How is a diet that high in saturated fat possibly going to make you healthy?

Your patients are not getting that message, but it's what they need to hear.

TREATING CERAMIDES

One of the best signs of how dangerous ceramide can be is the effort underway to develop drugs to stop the production of it. A lot of people are working to develop those drugs. The effort is analogous to the development of drugs to treat high cholesterol. Researchers think that if they can develop a drug that blocks ceramide production in people with a predisposition to accumulating this toxic fat, they can prevent type 2 diabetes and other metabolic conditions in those people.

I suspect these drugs could be highly beneficial, and for older patients, they could be lifesaving. That's good, but drugs should not be a free pass to eat as much saturated fat as you want or to forgo exercise. Instead, these drugs should be a backstop for when diet and exercise are not enough to lower ceramide and cholesterol. There are patients who can't control cholesterol or ceramide production with diet and exercise, but they are rare.

The primary method for reducing ceramide is to replace saturated fat calories with starchy carbohydrate calories that are unrefined. I don't recommend replacing saturated fat with polyunsaturated fat calories but instead with whole grains, potatoes, sweet potatoes, corn, beans, lentils, and rice—the kind of foods humans ate for thousands of years without epidemics of metabolic disease.

The evidence against ceramide is solid; you do not want high circulating levels of ceramide. The evidence that shows reducing saturated fat reduces ceramide levels is also incredibly strong.[148] [149] [150] Patients who reduce their saturated fat intake also get the added benefit of lowering their cholesterol.

ADVISING YOUR PATIENTS

It's true that more research into ceramides is needed, but that doesn't mean patients and medical professionals should wait to act. We already know that ceramide causes insulin resistance in the liver, so we don't need a long scientific explanation of that process to advise our patients to cut saturated fat from their diet. We already know that ceramide causes beta cell dysfunction in the pancreas, so we don't need to produce a hundred scientific studies before we can tell patients what to avoid eating. We know ceramide kills cardiac cells, but the precise scientific explanation isn't needed before we talk to our patients about their diet.

There is more than enough evidence to compel us to act. It took us a hundred years to reach a consensus on cholesterol, but does that mean we wouldn't have saved lives by advising patients to reduce their cholesterol back when Nikolai Anitschkov first discovered the danger in the 1930s?

If someone had figured out during the Roman Empire that mosquitoes caused malaria and found a way to rid cities and towns of mosquitoes, millions of lives would have been saved. Nobody needed to know the scientific details about the microbes that mosquitoes carry when they bite people and how those microbes circulate through the body and damage red blood cells. This information is useless when it comes to controlling malaria because the most important component of controlling malaria is getting rid of mosquitoes.

Similarly, we already know enough about the dangers of cholesterol and ceramide to give our patients actions they can take immediately to reduce their levels of those fats and reduce their risk of heart attack, stroke, diabetes, and cancer. If you can keep your saturated fat consumption to

6 percent or less of your total daily calories, you kill most of the mosquitoes.

If you have a patient who has been thoroughly convinced by industry propaganda that they should no longer worry about cholesterol, you now have another arrow in your quiver.

"Okay, fine," you can say. "So you don't think cholesterol is bad. Well, here's *another* problem: ceramide. It's completely independent of cholesterol and not mediated by cholesterol. Yet it shows major metabolic harms and results from the exact same behaviors. So lower your saturated fat intake!"

We may need more research on ceramide, but we need *much* more research on how to get people to stop eating so much saturated fat.

While some scientists are turning their attention to the dangers posed by ceramide, others are looking at the risks posed to our neurological and brain health from a diet rich in saturated fat. If dietary fat can cause plaque to form in the arteries throughout our body, would it have any impact on the arteries feeding blood to our brain?

Unsurprisingly, yes. Read on to find out how.

Chapter 7

DEMENTIA

We know from a century of research, clinical trials, and metabolic ward studies that a diet high in saturated fat causes cardiovascular disease. We also know that cardiovascular disease has been associated with dementia because the plaque that constricts blood flow to the heart can also form in intracranial arteries and constrict blood flow to the brain. When we look at photos of the cerebral arteries in neurologically healthy people, they look clear and flexible. But the arteries of patients with Alzheimer's disease[151] are clogged with the same deadly, yellow plaque we see in heart attack victims.[152]

This is no coincidence.

The consensus of scientists who research dementia is that dementia is a vascular disease.[153] It is caused by the same physiological processes that cause vascular disease elsewhere in the body.[154]

In one study, researchers examined a group of patients in their fifties for the presence of vascular disease risk factors, including high cholesterol, smoking, high body mass index, high blood pressure, and diabetes. More than twenty years later, these same 346 dementia-free patients underwent positron emission tomography brain imaging to discern their levels in their brain of beta-amyloid—the protein associated with the development of Alzheimer's.

Previous studies had noted that vascular disease risk factors in midlife increased the risk of dementia later in life, but scientists weren't sure if the risk factors were directly associated with the accumulation of beta-amyloid in the brain.

But this study revealed that those who had two or more risk factors had significantly high levels of beta-amyloid. The more vascular risk factors, the more beta-amyloid. This solidified the connection between vascular disease and the development of Alzheimer's[155] and reinforced a 2007 study finding that vascular factors play a role in the development of dementia. What's more, a study in the Netherlands showed that people with severe atherosclerosis due to high cholesterol had a three-fold greater risk of developing Alzheimer's-type dementia. Even those with mild-to-moderate atherosclerosis were still at significantly higher risk than those without it.[156]

Alzheimer's, we must conclude, is a vascular disease.[157]

THE IMPACT OF ALZHEIMER'S

If dementia were the only thing caused by saturated fat, that would be enough for me to restrict it in my diet. I would not keep looking for another reason. Surveys show[158] that people fear dementia more than any other condition, including cancer, and I understand why. I've watched it take both of my grandmothers' and my father's lives.

Dementia is a devastating condition. Not only does the patient lose connection with the rest of the world, but the disease puts a staggering financial and emotional strain on those around the patient.

It was heart-wrenching to watch my grandmother not recognize my grandfather and doubly so to watch my father, who had a PhD in philosophy, unable to complete a children's crossword puzzle or remember the names of me and my siblings. I see families every day that are destroyed by this condition and go through the same struggles I went through.

The prevalence of dementia is on the rise in the United

States as our population gets older. There are an estimated 6 million people in our country afflicted with Alzheimer's, the most common type of dementia. Most of those—about 5.6 million—are sixty-five or older. By 2050, there could be nearly 14 million people suffering from Alzheimer's in our country. It is already the sixth-leading cause of death in the United States[159] and an increasing number of people in their late forties are being diagnosed with dementia.[160]

Scientists still aren't sure what precisely causes Alzheimer's disease. It is described in the ancient literature and seems to have been present for as long as humans have been around. We know part of it is genetic, but in all likelihood, it's a combination of genes, environment, and lifestyle choices, such as diet and exercise.

How big a part any one factor plays varies from patient to patient. Scientists have yet to find a drug that can influence the progression of Alzheimer's. They've tried nearly 150 different types, and while some drugs have helped reduce the sticky plaque that forms in the brain, none of the drugs has reversed the march of the disease once it's started. As a result, much of the research into the disease has shifted from treatment to prevention, and one of the most promising avenues for prevention focuses on getting people to reduce their consumption of saturated fat.

THE ROLE OF SATURATED FAT

Researchers are increasingly finding scientific evidence that a diet high in saturated fat attacks the brain in the same way it attacks the heart—by building a wall of plaque and restricting blood flow. As with most problems in the health field, though, it's often more complicated than that.

A small 2013 study[161] found, for example, that a diet high in saturated fat cuts the body's levels of apolipoprotein E, also called ApoE, which serves to guide amyloid beta proteins out of the brain. Left wandering around in the brain, amyloid beta protein forms plaque and has a greater likelihood of turning toxic in the brain. Researchers also found that patients on a high-saturated-fat diet had more amyloid beta in their spinal fluid.

The study didn't directly tie a high-saturated-fat diet to Alzheimer's because it wasn't extensive enough. But even those who noticed the limitations of the study admitted that it reinforced the idea that "taking good care of your heart is probably good for your brain too."[162]

While research into the causes of Alzheimer's and its relationship to a high-saturated-fat diet is ongoing, there has been enough scientific research to reveal a direct link between the amount of saturated fat in a person's diet and the likelihood that person will come down with Alzheimer's later in life. For example:

- Researchers found a correlation between Alzheimer's and elevated blood cholesterol.[163] Animals fed a high-fat and high-cholesterol diet had worse memories and learning capabilities than animals on a control diet. They lost more neurons and exhibited other Alzheimer's disease-related neuropathology. In Finland, a study involving more than 400 men found that those with elevated blood cholesterol in midlife had three times the risk of developing Alzheimer's.[164]
- Researchers followed a group of 815 healthy people over the age of sixty-five. Within about four years, 131 of those people had Alzheimer's, and researchers found that those who ate the most saturated fat had twice the risk of getting Alzheimer's. Diets high in unsaturated fats and unhydrogenated fats and low in saturated and trans fats seemed to protect against the disease.[165]
- In 2004, researchers noticed that patients who were taking statin drugs for high cholesterol had a significantly lower risk of developing Alzheimer's than a control group that didn't take the drug. Researchers weren't sure if there was something in the statin that provided the benefit or if the lower risk was merely related to lower cholesterol.[166]
- Some of the most compelling evidence that dietary fat is related to the development of Alzheimer's came from the Chicago Aging Study. Patients who had a diet high in saturated fat were twice as likely to

develop dementia, and even moderate consumption of trans fat, which has since been banned, increased the risk two to three times.[167]

- Researchers in another study in Rotterdam examined the diet and aging of more than 5,000 people fifty-five and older and found that those with a diet high in saturated fat and cholesterol increased their risk of dementia. However, consuming fish, a source of polyunsaturated fatty acids, may decrease the risk, researchers found.[168]

- Some studies have examined the value of vitamin E as a way to reduce the risk of Alzheimer's.[169] While the findings were not consistent from study to study, there is compelling evidence that getting vitamin E from vegetables, nuts, seeds (especially sunflower seeds), whole grains, and such fruits as avocados, apples, and melons provide antioxidant protection against Alzheimer's.

- In the Adventist Health Study, researchers studied nearly 3,000 residents of the Loma Linda, California, area and found that those who ate meat were twice as likely to become demented as those who were vegetarian.[170] When vegetarians developed Alzheimer's, it was often later in life than their meat-eating counterparts. Being vegetarian alone wasn't enough to protect my Adventist grandmother, who had a big bowl of ice cream every night while watching TV.

These findings align with what Dr. Alois Alzheimer

discovered in the early 1900s when he first described patients who were under sixty-five and getting dementia.[171] When he performed autopsies on these patients, he found massive build-ups of blood vessel plaque in their brains.

TREATING ALZHEIMER'S AND DEMENTIA

Although there have been several medications approved by the FDA to treat Alzheimer's, these medicines are mostly used to treat mild to moderate cases of the disease and really only address the symptoms. The physiological changes that lead to dementia take place unnoticed over many years, and once you become demented, there is no treatment for reversing the disease. Most of the drugs in use regulate neurotransmitters and help reduce symptoms or help with behavioral problems.

Eliminating saturated fat from your patients' diet isn't going to help them once they have Alzheimer's. But recommending they limit saturated fat early could go a long way toward preventing the disease later in life. Scientists are increasingly looking at the treatments used for cardiovascular disease and diabetes as possible interventions for dementia in patients.

Statin drugs used for lowering cholesterol are one of those interventions being examined. When I was in medical school, the predictions about the growth of Alzheimer's were pretty dramatic. Although the numbers are big and growing, they are not as bad as we once expected them to be because so many people have been treated for years with statin drugs to lower their cholesterol. They were given the drugs to prevent atherosclerosis, but the plaque in their intracranial arteries no doubt also benefitted.

When those of us in healthcare advise our patients, we can name several benefits to lowering their cholesterol. But one of the best reasons to reduce your cholesterol in your middle years is reducing your risk of spending your final years unable to recognize your family.

We've mentioned in earlier chapters that arterial plaque can't be removed and that is the consensus today among doctors and physiologists. Reducing a patient's blood cholesterol by 50 percent can shrink plaques, but only by 10 percent or so. Once it forms in the arteries of the heart or brain, plaque is generally there for good.

Or is it?

In primate trials, it's very clear that plaque can be reversed.[172] Scientists have taken New World monkeys and given them atherosclerosis on a high-saturated-fat diet. Then they have reversed that atherosclerosis by taking out all the saturated fat from their diet.[173]

We are also seeing good evidence from both drug and nutrition trials that atherosclerosis can be reversed. The best evidence comes from animal studies, but we also have some anecdotal and scientific evidence from humans. For example, the Lifestyle Heart Trial[174] led by Dr. Dean Ornish showed that intensive lifestyle changes, including exercise, meditation, diet changes, and emotional support, can reverse artery blockage and increase blood flow and function in the heart. There's no reason to think that can't also happen to the brain.

Then there is the case of Nathan Pritikin. He was diagnosed with severe atherosclerotic disease in the 1950s and put himself on an incredibly low-saturated-fat diet. He cut dairy, red meat, and eggs from his diet and took up running. His autopsy showed "near absence of atherosclerosis."[175]

TALKING TO PATIENTS

Patients, I've learned, do not like to talk about dementia. But if you're having a conversation with them about high cholesterol and you are discussing the dangers of consuming more than 6 percent of your calories as saturated fat, it makes sense to point to the connection between a high-fat diet and dementia later in life.

As a healer talking to patients about diet, you can point

to a growing list of frightening and life-altering risks that come from consuming too many saturated fats from dairy products, eggs, meat, fish, and tropical oils. If your patients are tired of hearing about heart disease, you can change the subject and point out how a diet high in saturated fat is also directly related to diabetes, ceramide, and dementia.

If your patient is young but showing signs of having consistently high cholesterol or any of these risk factors, the best choice you can help them make is to adopt a diet low in saturated fat. That means drastically reducing their consumption of high-fat dairy products like milk, cheese, and butter and drastically reducing or eliminating animal products and tropical oils from their menu. Tell them, "Let's deal with this now, before you develop severely clogged arteries and down the road have to deal with heart attacks, strokes, dementia, or all three."

If they need additional convincing, you can tell them the story about the folks in northern Finland. Not long ago, they were dying in droves from health problems brought on by their fatty, meaty diets. But they found a way to reverse that trend, and we'll explain how in chapter 8.

Chapter 8

WHEN COMMUNITIES CHANGE HOW THEY EAT

North Karelia is a far eastern province of Finland. It is a land of boreal forests where for generations people cut lumber for a living and lived off game, fish, berries, and the small number of root vegetables that grew well in the region's tough soils.

After World War II, when veterans were allotted small tracts of land as compensation for their service, people cleared their acreage and focused on raising livestock, including dairy cows that were known for producing milk with particularly rich fat content. With butter and dairy fat now prevalent, the North Karelia diet soon came to emphasize butter. Butter was in everything, from fish stew, which was half butter, to buttered potatoes and bread.[176]

By 1972, North Karelian men had the highest rate of heart attacks in the world.

The Finnish government was aware of the problem because North Karelia had been included in Ancel Keys' seminal Seven Countries Study.[177] Keys, the University of Minnesota physiologist whose work pointed to a connection between saturated fat and cardiovascular disease, and his colleagues had recruited nearly 13,000 middle-aged men from Finland, the United States, Japan, Italy, the Netherlands, Greece, and Yugoslavia for a long-term international study that began in 1958.

It was the world's first multicountry epidemiological study, and it focused on the relationship between diet and coronary heart disease and stroke. Keys hypothesized that the rate of coronary disease would vary according to dietary fat consumption and serum cholesterol levels.

Medical researchers in the Seven Countries Study poked, prodded, interviewed, and analyzed the diets and health of its subjects over the next twenty-five years, and a pattern quickly became apparent: the farther north you went, the more animal-based products people ate and the more often they developed heart disease.

The men in Greece and Italy, where plant-based diets dominated, rarely died of heart attacks. The two communities in Japan that were part of the study had similar mortality rates from coronary heart disease.

The biggest distinction among the 16 populations studied was between the Finns and the Japanese. While the Japanese got just 3 percent of their calories from saturated fat, the Finns got 22 percent, and the Finns' serum cholesterol levels were nearly twice that of the Japanese. Consequently, the Japanese had a death rate from coronary heart disease of around 5 percent while eastern Finland's death rate was 30 percent.[178] North Karelians, in particular, died on average ten years earlier and suffered thirty times as many heart attacks as men in Crete.[179]

Now, if the cholesterol deniers like Stephen Sinatra (the author of *The Great Cholesterol Myth*) were right, there would be no correlation between cholesterol and coronary heart disease in the Seven Countries Study. If diets high in saturated fat and low in carbohydrates were good for humans, then Finland would be one of the healthiest countries in Keys' research. But, in fact, the exact opposite is true.

Finland, embarrassed about the findings and worried about the health of its residents, initiated an aggressive public health campaign to convince North Karelians to change how they eat. (Americans *should* be embarrassed that we lose nearly more than half a million people annually to heart disease, because these are preventable deaths.) Finnish health officials launched an ad campaign, recruited hundreds of volunteer ambassadors to go from village to village to publicize the problem, and gave scores of public cooking classes demonstrating how to replace the butter and fatty pork in traditional stews with rutabagas, potatoes, and carrots.[180]

At the start of the project, coronary heart disease killed 670 North Karelians per 100,000 residents. Within ten years, that number had dropped by 33 percent, and by 2000, the death rate from coronary disease among middle-aged men in North Karelia had dropped an astonishing 73 percent. By then, the program had expanded throughout Finland, and the country's death rate from coronary disease among males aged thirty-five to sixty-four had dropped 66 percent. Average serum cholesterol levels, blood pressure, and smoking rates continue to decline as new generations of Finns see the value of adopting a diet low in saturated fat and animal products.[181]

We'll talk later in this chapter about how the North Karelians pulled this off, but for now we can say that North

Karelia is just one example of how communities haunted by vascular disease epidemics brought on by diets high in saturated fat can change and have changed in ways that give their citizens longer and higher-quality lives. North Karelia also illustrates how health officials can best communicate the need to make dietary changes and provide the tools people need to make those changes.[182]

THRIVING DURING TIMES OF WAR

Throughout recent history, we have examples of countries that by conscious choice or by the vagaries of war have had to change the average diet of their citizens. In some cases, war brings horrifying famine, such as those that struck Greece, Leningrad, and Java during World War II. From 1914 to 1918, more than 400,000 Germans died of malnutrition when the British blockaded the North Sea and prevented food shipments.

In other cases, however, food restrictions and shortages caused by war altered some countries' diet in a way that limited saturated fat and animal products in the average diet, leading to remarkable health improvements and lower death rates from noncommunicable diseases. Here are a few examples:

DENMARK IN WORLD WAR I

In 1917, Denmark, facing a World War I blockade, decided to de-emphasize protein in the national diet and turn more of its land over to grain production rather than livestock. Pigs and cattle were sold off, dairy production was reduced by 65 percent, and grains and potatoes were diverted from distillers and brewers to food makers.

The Danes, at the suggestion of Mikkel Hindhede, the manager of the Danish National Laboratory for Nutrition Research in Copenhagen and food advisor to the Danish government during World War I, switched from a diet heavy in meat to a diet comprised primarily of starchy grains and vegetables. The country came to rely on potatoes and barley. Barley previously grown for pigs now went to humans, and the menu in most homes during the blockade consisted of bran bread, barley porridge, potatoes, greens, and small amounts of milk and butter. Some farmers still had pork, but most of Denmark's 3 million citizens went without. A few rich people could afford beef.

Despite the blockade, Denmark's death rate dropped by 34 percent (!) while its neighbor Germany, which had focused on maintaining meat supplies, endured a devastating famine that led to the deaths of nearly half a million people. Denmark, which had remained neutral during the war, calculated that its reduced death rate meant that 6,300 lives had been saved during the war.

Hindhede is remembered as a hero for his recommendations to switch Danes to a plant-based diet, but the physician and nutritionist later wrote that he wasn't surprised by his success. "Since 1885, when I began my experiments with a low-protein diet (mostly vegetarian), I have been convinced that better physical conditions resulted from this standard of living," Hindhede wrote. "As the result of extensive studies in this field, I am convinced that overnutrition, the result of palatable meat dishes, is one of the most common causes of disease."[183]

NORWAY IN WORLD WAR II

Norway had a similar experience during World War II when the Germans occupied the country. The Germans diverted animal products and all calorie-dense foods to Germany, leaving the Norwegians to survive on fish, potatoes, and whatever vegetables they could grow. Norwegians during this time also smoked less and were more physically active, and as a result of these three changes, deaths from heart disease, stroke, and diabetes plummeted.

Norway has recently seen similar drops in heart attack deaths. The percentage of deaths from heart disease and cardiovascular disease dropped from 50 percent in 1975 to 33 percent in 2009. The number of heart attacks is as low as it was during World War II.

Doctors credit big drops in Norwegians' cholesterol levels, as well as better treatment, statin drugs, and beta blockers. Fewer people are smoking. Still, 70 percent of the population has high cholesterol, and the number of heart attacks among the young and middle-aged women has increased while the number among young and middle-aged men has decreased.[184]

UNITED KINGDOM IN WORLD WAR II

Something similar to Norway occurred in Britain during World War II when food was rationed.

Before the war, Britain imported much of its food, including 70 percent of its cheese and half of its meat. In 1940, the island nation began rationing butter, bacon, and sugar, and not long after began rationing meat, tea, jam, biscuits, breakfast cereals, cheese, eggs, lard, and milk. "Wholemeal" bread replaced the refined white bread most Brits enjoyed. The rationing continued for the next fourteen years. Bakers replaced fruit with carrots, and children considered carrots on sticks a special treat.[185]

As a result of these dietary restrictions, diabetes plummeted.[186] Although the rates soared again after the war when food supplies returned to normal, the generation that was subjected to rationing in their adolescent and early adult years came to be known as the "golden generation" or "golden cohort" for its ability to live longer, healthier lives than the generations on either side of them in history. Researchers aren't sure why those born between 1925 and 1934 have done so well, but they believe their rationed diets during the war years may have contributed. The wartime diet was rich in fruits and vegetables and low in saturated fat, and the British Office of National Statistics theorizes that diet "may have improved general health during childhood and later."[187]

CUBA IN THE 1990S

During the 1980s, Cuba under Fidel Castro received bountiful agricultural support from the Soviet Union, allowing Cubans to consume an average of 3,000–3,200 calories a day. In the early 1980s, the country's obesity prevalence was 12 percent but grew to nearly 15 percent by 1990. This was nowhere near the United States' current obesity rate of nearly 40 percent, but Cuba's obesity rate was higher than you'd expect from a largely rural, agrarian society like Cuba's in the 1980s.[188]

From 1991–1995, however, things changed. Cuba faced an economic crisis. The Soviet Union collapsed and its support to Cuba shriveled up. The US tightened its embargo on the island, preventing pharmaceuticals, manufactured goods, and food imports from entering the country. Food became more scarce, and gasoline was in short supply. Meat and dairy products were largely unavailable.[189]

Castro responded by ordering food rationing and eliminating most of the country's bus routes. He also encouraged Cubans to plant small-scale gardens to feed themselves until the country's large-scale agriculture could expand to meet the country's needs. The country stopped exporting as much sugar from sugar cane so Cubans could consume it as a stop-gap source of calories. Castro also acquired a million bicycles from China to distribute to Cubans who no longer had the option of riding the bus.

Cubans quickly adopted a vegan diet that included high fiber fresh produce, fruit, beans, corn, and rice. People ate what they could grow, catch, or pick. Smoking and drinking alcohol declined. With no gasoline for tractors, farmers tilled their fields with oxen teams and pulled weeds by hand. Cuba went organic.

As a result of lower calorie consumption and increased exercise, Cuba's obesity and heart disease rates plummeted. People lost an average of 12 pounds. The number of diabetes cases were cut in half, illustrating once again that sugar is not the primary cause of diabetes. The number of strokes and cases of cancer also declined. The political and economic difficulties Cuba faced during what Castro called "the special period" actually made Cubans healthier. In fact, they continued to go to work and school and carrying on as before. They just weren't as sick and fat as they had been before.

That all changed when the economy turned around. As meat, cheese, and processed foods became more available and cheaper, Cubans got fatter and exercised less. They ate more than they had before the crisis started. From 1995 to 2011, the country's obesity rate tripled and there was a 140 percent increase in diabetes. Diabetes mortality increased from 9.3 deaths per 10,000 people to 13.9 deaths in 2010. Deaths from heart disease returned to pre-crisis levels.[190]

When researchers from Spain, Cuba, and the US analyzed the nationwide statistics kept by the Cuban Ministry of Public Health, they recommended that "educational efforts, redesign of built environments to promote physical activity, changes in food systems, restrictions on aggressive promotion of unhealthy drinks and foods to children, and economic strategies such as taxation" are needed if countries want to improve the overall health of their citizens.[191]

There is a clear pattern when populations cut their consumption of saturated fat and replace it with starchy carbohydrates and a plant-based diet. These are not one-offs. There is nothing weird to explain. It's a clear-cut, obvious trend: when society drops its saturated fat consumption—either through necessity or by design—the number and rate of deaths from cardiovascular disease plummet.

These episodes from history have been thoroughly replicated on a smaller, more carefully controlled work from folks like Ornish and Dr. Caldwell Esselstyn, whose twelve-year research on heart disease showed that eliminating oil, dairy products, and all types of meat, including fish, arrested and reversed coronary athero-sclerosis. Esselstyn developed a diet based on the foods consumed in regions of the world that had little coronary disease and included lentils, grains, vegetables, fruit, and legumes. He put nearly 200 patients on that program, and of the 171 patients who stuck with it, only one had a vascular event. Of the twenty-one patients who dropped out of the diet, thirteen experienced a vascular event.

You don't need to take a statistics class to see that those results are significant.

IT TAKES HARD WORK

The North Karelia story spotlights the advantages of getting a large population to change its diet. But it also reveals the extraordinary effort required to make that change. This could be a valuable lesson for the United States, where governments are slow to enact dietary directives and the food industry is reluctant to accept irrefutable scientific findings if it threatens their producers' bottom line.

Let's take a closer look at what happened in Finland to see if we can tease some takeaways from their experience. What does it take to get so many people to drastically change their diet and lifestyle?

- **Public health officials focused on a noncommunicable disease (heart attacks) the same way they would address infectious diseases like flu epidemics or polio.** The Finnish Minister of Health saw heart disease as a terrifying public health crisis, an epidemic that needed to be addressed over a long period, and directed the necessary resources to attack it.
- **The project began with an ambitious public information campaign.** The government organized training events throughout the region, and students studied nutrition and the health issues related to diet in the classroom. Advertising and television programs that featured individuals getting their cholesterol measured created a stronger sense of community purpose.
- **The government enlisted nongovernmental**

organizations to help. The Martha Organization, an NGO that promotes home and family well-being, taught North Karelian women healthier ways to cook traditional recipes. Martha volunteers handed out recipe books that added vegetables to traditional stews that were previously made mostly with water, salt, and fatty pork. All told, more than 1,500 volunteers became ambassadors who gave talks to groups or dropped in on neighbors with information and demonstrations on cooking plant-based meals that tasted good.

- **Perkka Puska, the Finnish doctor who led the campaign in North Karelia, worked tirelessly to get food producers to make healthier products.** Puska knew he wouldn't make progress if healthy food wasn't readily available. But not surprisingly, food makers resisted. The dairy industry bought ads bashing the project and local sausage makers balked at reducing the pork fat and salt they used. But the ads backfired and led many citizens to accuse the dairy producers of purposely contributing to the problem. The sausage makers who reduced the pork and fat by adding mushrooms found that sales increased.

- **Although locally grown fruit was scarce, Puska convinced many dairy farmers to grow more blueberries, raspberries, and lingonberries.** The program also enlisted help from supermarkets, and when stores began to stock more frozen berries, year-round fruit consumption skyrocketed.

- **The program started small and grew.** The North Karelia Project was the first major community-based project aimed at preventing cardiovascular disease, and after the initial five-year project period showed promising results, the project expanded throughout Finland and internationally through the World Health Organization.
- **Healthcare providers were actively involved.** The project actively engaged with general practitioners and public health nurses in the campaign. Healers did not stand on the sidelines writing prescriptions for drugs but instead talked to patients about lifestyle choices and dietary changes that would improve their health. These patients, regularly exposed to the success stories of others, responded.
- **Vegetables became a thing.** Before the North Karelia Project, few people in the province ate vegetables or used vegetable oil, and 90 percent of the people put butter on their bread. By 2002, only 7 percent used butter that way and the mean serum cholesterol level in North Karelia had declined nearly 20 percent. The region's population had a high average blood pressure that was brought under control, and people reported spending more time doing physical activities. Life expectancy for men increased by seven years, and for women, it increased six years!

Puska's goal was to change "the whole system" rather than focusing on individual behaviors. North Karelia's culture resisted change, but everyone got involved—schools, health clinics, doctors and nurses, nonprofits, governments, food makers, grocery stores, and farmers—to reduce the consumption of saturated fat and increase consumption of a plant-based diet. The program also encouraged smokers to quit and for people to exercise more. "So much is known that the main question for (noncommunicable disease) prevention is not 'what should be done' but 'how should it be done,'" Puska wrote in a 2002 report for the World Health Organization.

Puska followed the advice of British epidemiologist Geoffrey Rose, who asserted that individual health reflected the overall population's health; if you could improve the community at large, individual gains are compounded. For example, Rose had shown that every percentage point you lowered a population's average cholesterol reading, you lowered heart disease in the population by two points. In his 2002 WHO report, Puska noted that reducing serum cholesterol levels in Finland has been the "strongest contributor" to decreases in the country's coronary heart disease.

Perhaps more importantly, the success of the North Karelia project highlights how preventing disease is more cost effective than treating diseases. As Dan Buettner notes in his book *The Blue Zones Solution: Eating and Living Like the World's Healthiest People*, healthcare in the United States—from doctors and hospitals to pharmaceutical companies—focuses largely on treating people after they're sick. North Karelia demonstrates what happens when you focus instead on keeping people from getting sick in the first place.

Finland gives us a great success story, but there are other examples of what happens when people make mistakes with their diet but survive and learn how to make changes. Read on to learn how they did this—and to gain tips for talking to your patients about changes they can make.

Chapter 9

TALKING TO YOUR PATIENTS

Bob Harper was the picture of health until he suffered a heart attack in 2017 and collapsed on the gym floor during a workout.

Harper is a personal trainer and one of the hosts of the TV show *The Biggest Loser.* He's fifty-three years old but looks much younger, particularly when he takes his shirt off. He's lean and muscular and is remarkably strong and fit for a man his age. But he would be dead today if a doctor at his gym hadn't used a defibrillator to restart his heart.

Although you don't hear him talk about it much, Bob Harper had high cholesterol. That's the only way to explain the type of massive heart attack he suffered. At the time of his collapse, Harper famously followed and promoted a paleo diet that was high in fat and protein and low in carbohydrates. From what we know about how a diet high in saturated fat increases serum cholesterol, it's no surprise that Harper suffered a massive heart attack.

Harper switched to a new eating plan—outlined in his weight-loss book *Super Carb Diet*—after his heart attack. The new diet emphasized healthy whole grains, including quinoa, brown rice, and whole-grain bread. He's cut red meat and eats fish and chicken instead. He admits the high-fat meals he used to endorse didn't do much for his heart.

Even with the dietary changes Harper has made, he still serves as a cautionary tale for people. Harper, despite his extreme level of fitness, had high cholesterol and an inherited risk of a heart attack, and if he had been put on a low-saturated-fat diet in his thirties, he probably never would have had a heart attack in the first place.

His story also underscores the fundamental problem about diet in our country: we have a food industry that doesn't care about health and a health industry that doesn't care about food. And we get exactly the results you would expect from those two facts, which is disastrously unhealthy food and disastrously poor health. Ninety percent of the problems people see their doctor about are metabolic problems caused by two things: diet and lifestyle. Yet doctors don't feel comfortable talking about either of those things.

We need to change that.

THE MESSAGE IS CLEAR

At this point in history, there is no chance that we will ever learn that high LDL cholesterol does not cause heart disease. We have a century's worth of solid proof. Let's be clear about that.

What's disappointing about the Bob Harper story is that even though he changed his diet and his dietary recommendations for the people who follow him, he still gives scant attention to the dangers of saturated fat. He doesn't make a strong enough connection between the health of his heart and all the saturated fat he was consuming at the time.

It's as if all of us have a collective amnesia that these relationships between dietary saturated fat and increased serum cholesterol can be described by an equation. (see "Keys' equation: Change in serum cholesterol concentration" in chapter 4.)

As healers, we need to use every opportunity we have to

make that connection for our patients. When we advised our patients about smoking, we told them to quit. A lot of people did quit, but even those who didn't probably cut back on their smoking somewhat after we counseled them. We need to take the same approach when it comes to dietary saturated fat; if we advise our patients to eliminate it from their diets, they will probably still consume some saturated fat, but the amount will be greatly reduced and they will enjoy major health benefits.

Harper, in many interviews he gave after his heart attack, blamed his coronary illness largely on lipoprotein(a), which increases your risk of heart attack or stroke. Lp(a) was a factor, no doubt, but it was also a convenient way for Harper to sidestep the role his diet played in clogging the arteries to his heart. Regardless of whether someone has the inherited Lp(a) trait, if their LDL is too high, they have to get it down. A genetic quirk doesn't absolve you from taking responsibility for high cholesterol.

Besides, you can reduce your Lp(a) with a diet that is low in saturated fat and high in plant fiber and complex carbohydrates.[192] Researchers at Georgia State and the University of Texas Health Science Center found that a plant-based diet reduced Lp(a) by 16 percent and LDL by 30 percent in about a month.[193]

Your genetics are like the make of your car. If you crash

head-on into a brick wall with a Volvo or a BMW, you're in much better shape than if you crash with an old AMC Gremlin. But isn't your best choice to avoid crashing in the first place? The evidence is incredibly strong that populations that eat plant-based diets low in saturated fat and keep their LDLs under the guideline numbers don't have heart disease at all. They don't get dementia at the high rates seen in Western countries. They might be driving genetic Gremlins, but they are steering away from the crash.

STRIKING THE RIGHT TONE

I'm not suggesting it's easy to talk to patients about their diet. In my current practice, patients often want to talk about their diet, but when I see patients for routine ailments, I find they can still take it personally when you talk to them about nutrition, especially if they have a weight issue. They think you are judging them, and when they sense that, the game is lost.

People are also frequently opaque about their diet. You can ask them what they typically eat and they generalize. They'll tell you they don't eat a lot of red meat or that they "eat healthy." A survey by *Consumer Reports* found that 90 percent of Americans think they have a healthy diet. The same survey found that only 11 percent of respondents felt they were overweight, even though the Centers for

Disease Control and Prevention estimates that nearly 70 percent of Americans are overweight or obese.

Clearly, there is a disconnect.

If you're having a discussion about diet with a patient, you may have to be a bit persistent so that you can break down their specific meal choices. If their cholesterol is 200, you're not going to hear that they have oatmeal for breakfast, broccoli and brown rice for lunch, and sloppy Joe's made with lentils for dinner. You'll hear something else, and if it's a vague response, you can assume it's a diet high in saturated fat and refined foods. When this happens, you may have to just tick off some foods they should avoid—candy, high-fat foods, grain-based desserts, fast food, and so forth. They may not tell you what they're eating, but they will start thinking more about what they are eating, and that alone will help them choose better.

Patients will also say they eat a lot of salad, like that is a good thing. It usually isn't. Coleslaw can be anything from sesame seeds and cabbage with a little vinegar to something that's basically mayonnaise with a bunch of wilted leaves in it. Both are called coleslaw but one is relatively healthy and the other is full of saturated fat. A McDonald's kale salad served in Canada has more calories than a Double Big Mac.[194]

You must be sensitive to the emotional aspect of a person's diet. For some people, food is a primary relationship in life. You have a generation of people in their forties and fifties who grew up eating Big Macs—something I'm sure McDonald's is aware of and has worked hard to foster. Avoid sounding preachy. At the same time, you can't validate the behavior and say, "Well, if you cut down to two Big Macs a week, that's okay," because it's not.

Since 30 percent of American patients are obese, you would expect there to be some conversation about diet in the exam room. Fifteen percent of people smoke, and when doctors find out a patient still smokes, they talk to the patient about the dangers. We expect that from our healthcare system. But when it comes to diet and saturated fat, which causes way more morbidity and disability than smoking, we fail to get the right message across. We should bring it up in every visit, just like we do with smoking.

To help you overcome that reluctance, here are some tips for talking to patients about saturated fats.

FEED THEM THE RIGHT NUMBERS

I recommend patients follow the American Heart Association guideline, which is that you should limit your calories from saturated fat to 6 percent or less of your total calories. If you're eating 2,000 calories a day—which is the average-sized person's target—that amounts to 120 calories per day from saturated fat, which is about 13 grams. It's also equal to about one slice of Daiya vegan cheesecake.

However, I think most people are better off consuming no added saturated fat. Most foods—even healthy vegetarian lentil soup in a can—will have some small amount of saturated fat in it. If your patients aim for zero, they're more likely to come in under that 6 percent limit, and they're more likely to see great results.

GET THEM TO EXERCISE

I recommend patients get into a regular exercise program unless they are quite obese with a body mass index over 35. In those cases, we try to get their diet under control, and as they start dropping weight, they can start exercising. If your patient is heavy and eating poorly, exercising too soon can be counterproductive because their risk of injury is so high. However, the patient's goal should be to get to a point where exercise is possible. Even those who are at a healthy weight should exercise—the metabolic, cardiac, neurological, bone health, and psychiatric benefits are well established.

Exercise alone doesn't cause weight loss, but any weight losses can't be sustained without regular exercise.

What isn't so well established is how to motivate all people to exercise, regardless of their current weight. Whoever figures that out should win the Nobel Prize. I encourage patients to do something they enjoy or to find something they enjoy. If you like to hike, go for hikes. If you love swimming, get a pool pass.

REFER THEM TO A REGISTERED DIETITIAN

Registered Dietitians (RDs) are more than happy to see patients and talk to them about diet. Not nearly enough people are being referred to dietitians. However, you must ensure the dietitian you are referring hasn't bought into the media narrative about how great fats are and how bad carbs are.

Even if you refer to an RD it's still imperative for doctors and other healthcare professionals to address the issue of saturated fat. When we find out a patient smokes, we don't merely hand them a referral slip to a smoking cessation clinic. No, we ask how much they smoke and how long they've been smoking, and we reinforce the dangers. Then we can send them to a smoking-cessation clinic with a greater hope they will follow through.

GIVE UP THE IDEA OF "CHEATING"

Most people aiming to cut saturated fat from their diet will fall off the wagon from time to time. When that happens, it's going to raise your serum cholesterol significantly and for longer than most people realize. Those high levels are going to persist for several days. When you compare two vegetarians, the one vegetarian who cheats and eats meat at one meal a week has significantly higher cholesterol than the other vegetarian who doesn't cheat.

It's important that your patients know that. Cheat meals undermine all their hard work from the past two weeks and leave them with a glut they have to work to reduce over the next two weeks. In this sense, one big cheat day can set you back for an entire month. Once that meal is consumed, there is nothing they can do to extract the fat and get a do-over. All they can do is redouble their efforts and get back on the wagon.

WHAT A MEDITERRANEAN DIET REALLY MEANS

The value of a plant-based Mediterranean diet has been well-documented, particularly in the Seven Countries Study we talked about in the last chapter. Bob Harper says he's adopted a Mediterranean diet.

If your patients mention going on a Mediterranean diet, make sure they don't modify it for their own tastes. If they throw in a lot of fats, oils, eggs, meat, and cheese, it's not a healthy Mediterranean diet. Fettucine alfredo with egg noodles and cream sauce with ossobuco and tiramisu for dessert is not going to lower LDL and reverse vascular disease.

And a trip to Italy doesn't mean you don't have to worry about your diet. Italians are increasingly forgoing their traditional diet of noodles, vegetables, and olive oil for a more Western diet that emphasizes red meat and butter. Less than half of Italians eat a traditional Mediterranean diet. As a result, obesity in Italy is on the rise, and more than a third of Italian children are either overweight or obese by the time they're eight.[195]

The Mediterranean doesn't typically eat this way anymore, so a trip to Italy for two weeks isn't going to lower your LDL.

BE CLEAR ABOUT WHAT THERAPEUTIC LIFESTYLE IS

The guidelines say you should allow three months of a therapeutic lifestyle before prescribing statins for someone with high cholesterol. Few doctors follow that three-month guideline when they have a patient with an LDL of 160 who declares they aren't changing *anything* about their lifestyle. You might as well break out the statins right away.

But if patients say they want to make changes, let them

know what that entails: exercise, weight loss, increased dietary fiber, decreased dietary fat, and reduced saturated fat. Those five things have been the standard recommendations since the 1970s. Don't let your patients get sidetracked by weird news reports that say something like high-fat cheese contains a crucial biomarker.

In a study of patients with prediabetes who were given those five goals, none of the patients who met four out of the five goals went on to develop type 2 diabetes.[196]

KNOW THE TOP FIVE SOURCES OF SATURATED FAT

Most medical providers should know this off the top of their heads when talking to patients. The top five sources are cheese; pizza; grain-based desserts like cookies, cakes, pies, and brownies; dairy-based desserts like ice cream, yogurt, and Frappuccino; and chicken.

Notice something interesting? All of the top four get most of their saturated fat from dairy products, tropical oils, or eggs. There may be a little meat on pizza, but it's dwarfed by the cheese and the grease in the dough (Pizza Hut, I'm looking at you). Yet hardly a week goes by that someone doesn't claim dairy products have beneficial effects of some sort, almost always funded by the dairy industry.

They even tried to claim chocolate milk helped with concussions![197]

As for chicken, when you compare it to other animal muscles, it isn't that high in saturated fat, but it makes the list because it's the most common single meat people eat. Chicken consumption in the US went up 600 percent in the 20th century. Hardly anyone could claim Americans got healthier during that time. If chicken were a health food, this shouldn't be the case.[198]

However, if "red meat" were listed as a single category, it would still be the largest source of saturated fats of the meats, so I do have to caution people to replace their chicken with chickpeas and not beef or pork.

When I'm counseling patients, I tell them to avoid all these foods high in saturated fat and replace them with healthy plant foods like potatoes, sweet potatoes, corn, peas, beans, lentils, and rice. When I have patients who do that, they lose weight—in some cases in just reducing their consumption of the top five—and I see improvement in all their biomarkers.

Banning the top five is a simple and cheap low-saturated-fat diet that anyone can explain in a short time.

IF THEY'RE ONLY WILLING TO MAKE ONE CHANGE...

Those of us in healthcare need to know that if there is only one thing you can get your patients to change, convince them to drop dairy. It's the single largest source of saturated fat in the American diet. And when I say 'drop dairy,' I mean giving up *all* dairy. I tell patients to look at the labels and see if there are any milk products in anything, since there are other components in dairy that have negative health effects.[199] [200] [201]

A few years ago there was a push for people to eat a "paleo diet." This diet eliminated grains and beans, which I don't recommend, but it also cut out dairy and some of the people who adopted it saw massive health benefits, potentially due to this.

I also advise them to give up anything that *looks* like dairy. Most dairy substitutes are trying hard to replicate the mouth feel and flavor effects that saturated fat adds to dairy products. Foods like Ben and Jerry's nondairy ice cream is made with coconut oil, and most vegan cheese is made with tropical oil. Most dairy replacement products have as much saturated fat as the dairy version. Don't just give up dairy, give up "dairy," including those things that look or act like mammalian milk byproducts. If you want something to pour on cereal, there are many acceptable nondairy milks that are low in saturated fat. You can also use these to make recipes that call for cow's milk.

AVOID RESTAURANTS, INCLUDING VEGAN RESTAURANTS

Patients need to realize that restaurants are a danger zone. The best way to get a good, low-saturated-fat meal in a restaurant is to turn the menu upside down and just ask the waiter to work with you. Whenever you're eating fast food or eating in a sit-down restaurant, you're going to get more saturated fat than you should. See if they have potatoes or bowls of rice you can have with your salad (hold the dressing and use lemon juice or vinegar without the oil).

Most vegan or vegetarian restaurants will be lower in saturated fat, but not by much because of all the tropical oils they use. These restaurants are in a tough spot, they are trying to convince people who normally eat an unhealthy diet to try something less unhealthy but which has the same hedonic pleasure and mouthfeel that they're used to. That's a difficult order to fill.

Some vegan restaurants do work to have menu items available for people trying to limit total and saturated fats, but I advise patients looking to reverse health conditions to ask lots of questions about the food before they order. The restaurant can't stay open if they don't get repeat business, so their primary goal is food that Americans will think is tasty, which usually means substantial use of unhealthy fats.

BE MINDFUL OF VITAMIN B12

All healthcare providers who advise people to reduce their saturated fat must be sure the patients have a good source for vitamin B12. Vitamin B12 deficiency increases your risk of heart disease and neurological disorders. It can also give you nerve damage.

People who are trying to eat a healthy diet should be regularly tested for B12 deficiency. Even if you're not deficient, use a daily supplement. You don't want to wait until you're deficient.

Any patient who is over fifty, has a gastrointestinal absorption problem, or takes Metformin, a proton pump inhibitor, or an H2 blocker should also take a supplement, since these can all make you B12 deficient.

FITNESS ALONE CANNOT BE ENOUGH

Harper, in the years since his heart attack, has used his bully pulpit to send some good messages. He's promoted a diet focused on unrefined, fiber-rich carbs. His new recipes allow for too much fat, from my point of view, but he's also talked about the dangers posed by his former diet, which was much higher in fat. He's also called attention to the risk heart patients face of having another cardiac episode. One in four heart attacks in the United States is suffered by someone who has already had at least one event.

Harper's story is similar to what happened to Jim Fixx, the author of *The Complete Book of Running,* which has been credited with helping start a fitness revolution in the 1970s. Fixx and other writers who ran long distances thought our increasingly industrialized culture was causing the country's epidemic of heart disease, and they prescribed running as the cure. People should listen to their bodies, not their doctors, Fixx thought.

Fixx died in 1984 at the age of 52 while out on a run near his home in Vermont. At the time of his death, atherosclerosis had almost entirely blocked two coronary arteries. A third was 70 percent blocked. He ran through chest pain and discomfort but refused to see u doctor.

What message can we glean from the stories of Jim Fixx and Bob Harper? Some might see them as an excuse not to take up running or cross-fit, Harper's preferred workout, but that's missing the point. The point is this: diet matters. Harper ate a paleo diet. Fixx loved fast food and donuts. They were both remarkably fit and trim individuals but their diets delivered too much cholesterol to their bloodstream and their hearts failed as a result.

In 1984, Fixx called Nathan Pritikin, a runner and persistent advocate for using low-fat diets to treat clogged arteries, to complain about Pritikin's book, *Diet for Runners.* In particular, Fixx thought Pritikin's chapter "Run and Die on the American Diet" was "hysterical" and would frighten a lot of runners. Pritikin said that was his intent. Pritikin *wanted* to frighten runners into taking up a low-fat diet.

"I think it's better to be hysterical *before* someone dies than after (emphasis added)," Pritikin told Fixx. "Too many (people) have already died because they believed that anyone who could run a marathon in under four hours and who was a nonsmoker had absolute immunity from having a heart attack."

Fixx, sadly, believed otherwise, and six months later, he was dead from a heart attack.

I understand that even well-informed and knowledgeable healthcare professionals aren't going to be able to convince all their patients to change. All we can do is be clear and persistent about the messages we send our patients. If your patients are overwhelmed with confusion about what to eat and what to avoid and whether the caveman diet is better than the Atkins Diet, concede that they have a right to be. It *is* confusing.

The medical advice on smoking was confusing until the 1980s. Until that time, some doctors recommended switching cigarette brands or reducing consumption to under ten cigarettes a day. We now realize that was ridiculous advice.

Patients need to understand that there is no chance that next week someone's going to come out with a legitimate study showing saturated fat in your diet is good for you. It can't happen. The evidence to the contrary is simply too powerful, and one of the most effective ways to help people understand that is for healthcare professionals like you and me to become more forceful about telling them.

CONCLUSION

GETTING EVERYONE ON
THE SAME PAGE

It's never easy talking to patients about their diet. Getting people to change how they eat is about as easy as getting them to change the relationships they're in. Just as you have an emotional attachment to your relationship, you have an emotional attachment to your food.

Many patients are uncomfortable with the subject, and many of us in the healthcare field are confused about what to say. We are often subjected to the same doubts our patients have because the food industry tries to manipulate the science.

But that's no reason why we shouldn't play a central role in getting our country to turn its health around the way the folks in North Karelia did, or the way the folks in Denmark did during World War I, or the way the people of the Mediterranean have done up until recently.[202]

Our job may be to treat people who are sick, but the best way to do that is to prevent them from getting sick in the first place. Remember, we want to have a fence blocking people from falling rather than giving them exquisite Pillow Top mattresses at the bottom of the cliff.

When we look at the soaring rates of cardiovascular disease, diabetes, dementia, cancer, and stroke, there is one thread that runs through it: saturated fat. This is not a theory. It is not controversial, no matter how much media reports try to make it seem so. It's been proven scientifically so many times that it seems like a waste of time to continue debating it or even studying it.

A diet that has more than 7 percent of its calories coming from saturated fat is dangerous. The average American gets nearly 20 percent of their calories from trans fat and saturated fat[203]—nearly three times the maximum recommended amount. That's good news for the pizza chains and the milk and cheese producers. The beef industry should be happy, as well as the fast-food industry. But it's bad news for those of us who have made it our life's work to help people live longer, healthier, and productive lives.

In the ten-plus years since the worldwide dairy industry met in Mexico City, we've all heard a steady stream of noise that cheese, dairy products, and saturated fat are not nearly as bad as we all thought. That noise continues up to today, with "research" articles paid for by the industry coming out at least once a month saying that saturated fat isn't a problem. Other media outlets pick up the "news" in a feed-forward loop. The industry doesn't go so far as to say their products are *good* for people, but that's what people hear. They don't hear about the countless studies that show the damage that high levels of saturated fat in your diet will wreak.

We need a sea change in our attitude toward saturated fats.

BEING BLUNT ABOUT THE DANGER

We've seen this kind of sea change in society before. I remember in the seventies when it was nearly impossible to get away from cigarette smoke. People smoked in restaurants, at work, and on airplanes. People became worried about their health and the health of their children. No parent wanted their children to suffer the same problems they saw in their friends who smoked. They demanded change—and they got it. Getting the ball rolling was the most important thing. The more places that became tobacco-free, the easier it became to get even more places tobacco-free.

The same thing could happen if people became more aware of the facts about their diet and the fat in the products they buy at the grocery store. We can help them build that awareness. When something is directly linked to disease the way the typical diet is, healthcare providers have a responsibility to be blunt with patients and make clear, unequivocal recommendations about how their patients should eat.

Let's say the problem wasn't an epidemic of cardiovascular disease caused by diet but instead was the problem of too many people crashing their cars into walls at high rates of speed. If you advocated for safer cars and reductions in speed—the same way you might advocate lowering a person's LDL cholesterol—you could save a lot of lives.

But did you solve the problem? Even if you were successful getting better-built autos and reducing speed, you'd still have people driving into walls and dying. People would still suffer horrific deaths, and the only way to stop that is to get rid of cars altogether. If we got everyone to buy a Volvo and drive less than 35 mph, a lot fewer would die but some still would. The best way to stop the problem is to stop crashing altogether.

The best solution would be cars that simply can't crash, which technology is making more and more possible.

Most new cars by 2020 will have collision detection that automatically brakes the car when it senses an impending crash. This is what we need in healthcare for heart disease, dementia, diabetes, and stroke—an automatic alarm system that warns people of a major health issue so they can take action to stop it.

THE WORLD OF COKE

If you think the food industry has damaged Americans' health by promoting high-fat, processed, and sugary products, consider what it's doing in places like China.

Although the Chinese faced food shortages just a few decades ago, today 42 percent of the adults in China are overweight or obese and 20 percent of its children are obese, thanks largely to the processed foods that have flooded the country since it reformed its market economy and invited Western food companies to do business there.[204] Now giant Western food companies like Coca-Cola, Nestle, McDonald's, Pepsi Co., and Yum! Brands have not only reshaped the Chinese diet, but they also have a hand in formulating public health policies in China and other countries.[205]

Coke and its cohorts have formed a group called the International Life Sciences Institute, which works to stave off food regulation and soda taxes in China, Mexico, South Africa, India, and Brazil. The trade group is so well-entrenched that it shares offices with China's Centre for Disease Control and Prevention in Beijing and has seventeen branches in emerging economies around the world.

As a result, public health campaigns in those places promote exercise as a way to control weight but say little about the dangers of eating too much fatty junk food and sugary beverages. In early 2019, the *Journal of Public Health Policy* revealed why: Since 1999, Coke's faux research institute has "redirected China's chronic obesity disease science, potentially compromising the public's health." With Coca-Cola's help, the Chinese decided that the best way to solve its burgeoning obesity dilemma is to get children to exercise for ten minutes a day. No need to prattle on about the dangers of high-calorie junk food.

The expansion of Western foodstuffs in emerging economies comes as soda sales in the US plummet and restrictions in the US—such as New York City's proposed ban on large drink sizes—become more common. Coke didn't want the same kind of regulatory angst in China, so it convinced the government there that exercise is what moves the obesity needle down, not improved diets. China's Ministry of Health's obesity prevention and management guidelines were actually written by the China office of the Life Sciences Institute.[206]

When Coke tried something similar in the US—enlisting the help of sympathetic scientists and forming a nonprofit called the Global Energy Balance Network to promote exercise rather than better diets—the media spotted the conflict of interest and blew the whistle. The network was abandoned in 2015[207] but Coke continued to influence science and health research in countries like China, where the state-run media don't ask as many pesky questions.

A CONSISTENT MESSAGE

As individual healthcare practitioners, we won't be facing off in a debate with the food industry. But we do need to be consistent about our advice to patients:

- **Complex carbohydrates should be the primary source of calories.** Highly refined carbohydrates like those in packaged snack food are not healthy, but complex carbohydrates from unrefined starch sources like potatoes, sweet potatoes, whole grains, beans, lentils, and rice are good for you. The average American should consume five to ten times more fruits and vegetables than they currently are.
- **Saturated fat is dangerous.** Everyone should strictly limit their intake of saturated fat to 6 percent or less of their total calories if they are at high risk of vascular disease and dementia (which is everyone). Swapping saturated fat with complex starchy carbohydrates

or whole-food sources of polyunsaturated fat significantly reduces a person's risk of cardiovascular disease.[208]

· **Industry-funded studies have a built-in conflict of interest.** Next time you read about a new study extolling the virtues of a high-fat diet rich in butter, cheese, meat, and tropical oils, find out who funded the study. If the food industry is behind it, or if it's not specifically refuting long-established equations linking saturated fat to high cholesterol, you should be skeptical of the results.

These three statements are backed by decades of basic science and observational epidemiology. In addition, multiple human trials and metabolic ward experiments have shown completely consistent results with the basic science and observational epidemiology. Experiments done on our closest relatives, the primates, have shown a direct reversible link between diets high in saturated fat and vascular disease.[209] A hundred and fifty years ago, it was rare for someone to die of cardiovascular disease. Today, about 610,000 Americans die each year from heart disease.[210] That's one in every four deaths. It's an epidemic.

How many of those heart attacks could have been prevented if we'd done a better job of warning our patients early about the dangers of high cholesterol and saturated fat? If counseling patients to reduce their intake of saturated fats reduced heart disease by only 30 percent, it would save more lives than almost any other single public health intervention. That's conservative. If we started on people in their twenties and really harangued the way we do about smoking, we would drop it by 60 or 70 percent. Our goals are too small. We are accepting too much. We should be embarrassed that so many die from a largely preventable disease.

GETTING THE WORD OUT

Turn on any football game and there's a parade of ads for Applebee's, Arby's, Burger King, Chili's, Denny's, Dairy Queen, IHOP, McDonald's, Outback, Pizza Hut, Red Lobster, Sonic, Taco Bell, and Wendy's. Open any magazine and you'll see famous people wearing a milk mustache or full-page ads proclaiming the amazing power of cheese or the incredible edible egg. You'll see all these foods that are so high in saturated fat but are so profitable to so many industries that the government sees fit to fund programs that increase their consumption.[211]

In the meantime, our patients suffer and die needlessly. The truth about saturated fat is getting drowned out by the loud voices of people who advocate healthier versions of our standard diet or high-fat, low-carb diets like Atkins. Bloggers and podcast hosts who tout the value of high-fat foods while taking money from "healthy" potato chip companies that fry their product in tropical oils add to the confusing din. If you want to know how much money there is in low-carb diets, consider how Mark Sisson sold his paleo dressing company, Primal Kitchen, to Kraft Heinz for $200 million.[212]

People hear these confusing messages that prevent them from fully grasping just how devastatingly strong the scientific case against saturated fat is.

We must be confident and forthright in the face of that disingenuous din. When we go into an exam room and hear a patient say, "I was told I should put coconut oil in my coffee to make me healthier," we have to confidently and without hesitation tell our patient that coconut oil is high in saturated fat and is definitely something they should avoid.

We also need to push against black-and-white thinking in nutrition. People can improve their health without being either completely low carb or eating a very, very high carbohydrate diet. Eating a potato chip or a small amount of oil won't hurt anyone whose overall eating pattern is acceptable. But we shouldn't give license to people to engage in bad habits. Diet is a continuum, and movement toward a healthier diet has benefits even when that movement isn't directly and immediately to perfection.

There's a healthy middle ground, and we should guide people in the direction to reduce saturated fat and focus on a healthy, plant-based diet.

Imagining, like Pollyanna, that just talking to your patient about saturated fat will get them to immediately quit eating it is silly. We know from all our attempts to change patients' behaviors that we won't get through to everyone. Anyone who gives advice for a living is used to it being ignored. The definition of good advice is not that patients will follow it perfectly but that if they did follow it perfectly it would benefit them.

It's critical that we talk to our patients about saturated fat, and it's necessary that we do it repeatedly. This is not something you can mention once and then forget about. It should be an ongoing topic of discussion, particularly for people who are already trying to reverse a disease or who are clearly on the road to developing a disease.

Those of us in lifestyle medicine who recommend diets very low in saturated fat see dramatic reversals of chronic diseases. Many cancers have spread too far or are too aggressive to reverse with lifestyle. If someone is already on dialysis, you're not going to bring their kidneys back. Somebody who has type 1 diabetes is never going to get pancreatic beta cells back until they can get a transplant or cell modification treatment working. Somebody who's demented can't regrow all their brain cells, and even if they did, those cells would have to learn all the stuff that the dead cells forgot. But if patients are not that far gone, they almost always recover significantly when they adopt a diet very low in saturated fat.

Life has a 100 percent mortality rate. No patient should be under the illusion that there's any one thing they can do to make themselves bulletproof. At the same time, someone in a war zone should know that bulletproof vests exist and decide whether they want to wear one or not.

Everyone needs to know that you can substantially reduce your chances of having a serious health problem by adopting a diet that's very low in saturated fat.

We know all the mechanisms. We have the data. We have the epidemiological data, the randomized controlled trial data, the case series data, and the individual patient data. They all show the same pattern. How much more do we need to know?

Consilience is when evidence from independent, unrelated sources converge on a strong conclusion.[213] There is consilience around the dangers of saturated fat. Across the spectrum of research, history, and geography, the conclusions have been consistent: a diet high in saturated fat can shorten your life and leave you sick in a variety of ways.

The only contrary voices come from a handful of researchers willing to take money from the dairy or egg industry or journalists who want you to buy their fat-praising books and who are paid by groups sympathetic to the animal agriculture industry.

This job is not easy or simple, but the message can be simple: we can prevent most cases of the number-one cause of death in the world by getting people to reduce their saturated fat and lower their LDL.

One of the best ways to get that message across is to adhere to it ourselves. It starts with us. Remember, patients didn't really stop smoking until they noticed that their doctors had quit.[214] [215]

In the same way we need to be consistent with the advice we are giving our patients. If they walk past the breakroom and see cheeseburger wrappers and empty Krispy Kreme boxes, they are going to discount any advice we give them in the exam room about eating healthy. Just like they did when we advised them to stop smoking and they noticed an ashtray on your desk. We, as healthcare providers, established the tone about smoking then and we have to do it again on the issue of saturated fat.

Nothing in life that's really worth doing is easy and getting patients and ourselves to change how we eat won't be either. But I hope reading this book has given you enough information to know that it will be worth it.

ABOUT THE AUTHOR

DR. EVAN ALLEN is a family practitioner and a third-generation vegetarian. He opened his private practice, Total Care Family Practice, in Henderson, Nevada, in June 2007. Prior to that, Dr. Allen was director of primary care at Fremont Medical Centers. He earned his medical degree from Loma Linda University Medical School and completed his residency through UC Davis at Travis Air Force Base in Fairfield, California. He was stationed at Nellis Air Force Base, achieving the rank of Air Force major before leaving the military to work in various clinics in southern Nevada. At Total Care, Dr. Allen provides a range of services, from physicals to weight loss to treating noncommunicable diseases. He is a member of the American College of Lifestyle Medicine and has received board certification by the American Board of Obesity Medicine. Dr. Allen enjoys watching sports, spending time with his son, playing racquetball, and studying biology, psychology, linguistics, philosophy, and history.

NOTES

1   Dr. John McDougall, "Denis Burkitt, MD Opened McDougall's Eyes to Diet and Disease," *The McDougall Newsletter*, January 2013. https://www.drmcdougall. com/misc/2013nl/jan/burkitt.pdf.

2   Apo(b)s, or apolipoprotein b, are proteins found in the lipoproteins that transport cholesterol through your bloodstream. Apo(b)-containing lipoprotein particles are the most damaging to our arteries. They contain not only LDL but also very low-density lipoproteins and chylomicrons—all three of which promote atherosclerosis.

3   Sacks, Frank M., Alice H. Lichtenstein, Jason HY Wu, Lawrence J. Appel, Mark A. Creager, Penny M. Kris-Etherton, Michael Miller et al. "Dietary fats and cardiovascular disease: a presidential advisory from the American Heart Association." *Circulation* 136, no. 3 (2017): e1-e23. https://www.ahajournals. org/doi/full/10.1161/CIR.0000000000000510.

4   Axelsson, Alf, and Fredrik Lindgren. "Is there a relationship between hypercholesterolaemia and noise-induced hearing loss?" Acta oto-laryngologica 100, no. 5-6 (1985): 379-386, https://www.tandfonline.com/doi/ abs/10.3109/00016488509126561.

5   Esposito, Katherine, F. Giugliano, Marco De Sio, D. Carleo, C. Di Palo, M. D'armiento, and Dario Giugliano. "Dietary factors in erectile dysfunction." *International journal of impotence research* 18, no. 4 (2006): 370. https://www. nature.com/articles/3901438.

6   Shamloul, Rany, and Hussein Ghanem. "Erectile dysfunction." The Lancet 381, no. 9861 (2013): 153-165. https://www.sciencedirect.com/science/article/pii/ S0140673612605200.

7   Scott, Alex, Johannes Zwerver, Navi Grewal, Agnetha de Sa, Thuraya Alktebi, David J. Granville, and David A. Hart. "Lipids, adiposity and tendinopathy: is there a mechanistic link? Critical review." *Br J Sports Med* 49, no. 15 (2015): 984-988. https://bjsm.bmj.com/content/49/15/984?int_source=trendmd&int_medium=trendmd&int_campaign=trendmd.

8   Kauppila, Leena I., Raija Mikkonen, Pekka Mankinen, Kia Pelto-Vasenius, and Ilkka Mäenpää. "MR aortography and serum cholesterol levels in patients with long-term nonspecific lower back pain." *Spine* 29, no. 19 (2004): 2147-2152. https://journals.lww.com/spinejournal/Abstract/2004/10010/MR_Aortography_and_Serum_Cholesterol_Levels_in.12.aspx.

9   Marshall, J. A., D. H. Bessesen, and R. F. Hamman. "High saturated fat and low starch and fibre are associated with hyperinsulinaemia in a non-diabetic population: the San Luis Valley Diabetes Study." *Diabetologia* 40, no. 4 (1997): 430-438. https://link.springer.com/article/10.1007/s001250050697.

10 Kalmijn, Sandra, Lenore J. Launer, Alewijn Ott, Jacqueline CM Witteman, Albert Hofman, and Monique MB Breteler. "Dietary fat intake and the risk of incident dementia in the Rotterdam Study." Annals of neurology 42, no. 5 (1997): 776-782. https://onlinelibrary.wiley.com/doi/abs/10.1002/ana.410420514.

11 Phillips, Catherine M., Emmanuelle Kesse-Guyot, Ross McManus, Serge Hercberg, Denis Lairon, Richard Planells, and Helen M. Roche. "High dietary saturated fat intake accentuates obesity risk associated with the fat mass and obesity-associated gene in adults." The Journal of nutrition142, no. 5 (2012): 824-831. https://academic.oup.com/jn/article/142/5/824/4630756.

12 Kopelman, P. "Health risks associated with overweight and obesity." *Obesity reviews* 8 (2007): 13-17. https://onlinelibrary.wiley.com/doi/full/10.1111/j.1467-789X.2007.00311.x.

13 Hooper L, Martin N, Abdelhamid A, Davey Smith G. Reduction in saturated fat intake for cardiovascular disease. Cochrane Database of Systematic Reviews 2015, Issue 6. Art. No.: CD011737. DOI: 10.1002/14651858.CD011737

14 ENC Research Grants, Egg Nutrition Center, https://www.eggnutritioncenter.org/grant-fellowship/.

15 Tanja K Thorning, Farinaz Raziani, Nathalie T Bendsen, Arne Astrup, Tine Tholstrup, Anne Raben, Diets with high-fat cheese, high-fat meat, or carbohydrate on cardiovascular risk markers in overweight postmenopausal women: a randomized crossover trial, The American Journal of Clinical Nutrition, Volume 102, Issue 3, September 2015, Pages 573-581, https://doi.org/10.3945/ajcn.115.109116.

16 Julia Belluz, Vox Media, Food companies distort nutrition science. Here's how to stop them. https://www.vox.com/2016/3/3/11148422/food-science-nutrition-research-bias-conflict-interest.

17 During the nineteenth century, diabetes was rare in Ireland. There were 0.22 deaths from diabetes for every 100,000 people in 1840. That rate skyrocketed from 1880 to 1911 as fat and sugar consumption increased, and by 1972 there were 13.2 deaths from diabetes per 100,000 people, according to The Ulster Medical Journal from October 1987.

18 Crawford, E. M. "Death rates from diabetes mellitus in Ireland 1833—1983: a historical commentary." The Ulster Medical Journal 56, no. 2 (1987): 109.

19 NCD Risk Factor Collaboration. "Trends in adult body-mass index in 200 countries from 1975 to 2014: a pooled analysis of 1698 population-based measurement studies with 19.2 million participants." The Lancet 387, no. 10026 (2016): 1377-1396.

20 Zhang, Ronghua, Zhaopin Wang, Ying Fei, Biao Zhou, Shuangshuang Zheng, Lijuan Wang, Lichun Huang et al. "The difference in nutrient intakes between Chinese and Mediterranean, Japanese and American diets." Nutrients 7, no. 6 (2015): 4661-4688.

21 Brady Ng, "Obesity: the big, fat problem with Chinese cities." The Guardian, https://www.theguardian.com/sustainable-business/2017/jan/09/obesity-fat-problem-chinese-cities.

22 Gordon-Larsen, Penny, Huijun Wang, and Barry M. Popkin. "Overweight dynamics in Chinese children and adults." Obesity Reviews 15 (2014): 37–48.

23 Centers for Disease Control and Prevention, "Diarrhea: Common Illness, Global Killer," https://www.cdc.gov/healthywater/pdf/global/programs/globaldiarrhea508c.pdf.

24 The real molecule that causes problems, we now know, is a molecule called Apo(b). But because over 90 percent of the Apo(b) in anyone's serum is LDL, for the most part they measure the same thing. Since we have put decades of work into teaching patients about LDL, it still makes sense to focus on LDL rather than Apo(b).

25 Briggs, Robert D., M. L. Rubenberg, R. M. O'neal, W. A. Thomas, and W. S. Hartroft. "Myocardial infarction in patients treated with Sippy and other high-milk diets: an autopsy study of fifteen hospitals in the USA and Great Britain." Circulation21, no. 4 (1960): 538-542.

26 Carole Davis and Etta Saltos, "Dietary Recommendations and How They Have Changed Over Time, the US Department of Agriculture." https://www.ers.usda.gov/webdocs/publications/42215/5831_aib750b_1_.pdf.

27 Daniel, Carrie R., Amanda J. Cross, Corinna Koebnick, and Rashmi Sinha. "Trends in meat consumption in the USA." *Public health nutrition* 14, no. 4 (2011): 575-583.

28 A 2010 study published in Public Health Nutrition found that the US consumption of red meat has declined slightly since its peak in the late 1960s. The consumption of poultry has climbed steadily since the 1940s, and though it is still less popular than red meat, it is still the fifth highest source of saturated fat in the US diet, just ahead of a group including sausage, franks, and bacon. Red meat is not more prominent on the National Institutes of Health list because, unlike chicken, the NIH ranks it according to the various dishes red meat comes in. For example, burgers are seventh on the list and beef and beef mixed dishes are number nine.

29 Joseph, Abraham, Douglas Ackerman, J. David Talley, John Johnstone, and Joel Kupersmith. "Manifestations of coronary atherosclerosis in young trauma victims—an autopsy study." Journal of the American College of Cardiology 22, no. 2 (1993): 459-467.

30 Anonymous, "The Journalist Gary Taubes 2: A Parajournalism Paradox," PLANTPOSITIVE: Making the Case for Plant-Based Nutrition, http://plantpositive.com/2-the-journalist-gary-taubes-2/.

31 Even before Seven Countries Study, the research on saturated fat was strong enough that the American Heart Association used TV time in 1956 to warn people that a diet rich in butter, lard, eggs, and beef would lead to coronary heart disease. Despite these warnings, the United States government waited until the late 1970s to recommend that people adopt a low-fat diet in order to avoid heart disease.

32 National Institutes of Health, division of Cancer Control & Population Sciences, https://epi.grants.cancer.gov/diet/foodsources/sat_fat/sf.html.

33 Retterstøl, Kjetil, Mette Svendsen, Ingunn Narverud, and Kirsten B. Holven. "Effect of low carbohydrate high fat diet on LDL cholesterol and gene expression in normal-weight, young adults: A randomized controlled study." *Atherosclerosis* 279 (2018): 52-61.

34 Millen, Barbara E., Steve Abrams, Lucile Adams-Campbell, Cheryl AM Anderson, J. Thomas Brenna, Wayne W. Campbell, Steven Clinton et al. "The 2015 dietary guidelines advisory committee scientific report: development and major conclusions." *Advances in nutrition* 7, no. 3 (2016): 438-444.

35 For a comprehensive takedown of the entire low carb corpus, you can read Guyenet's notes on his recent debate with Taubes. http://www.stephanguyenet.com/references-for-my-debate-with-gary-taubes-on-the-joe-rogan-experience/.

36   Mary Ellen Shoup. "Pizza Hut adds 25% more cheese to pan pizzas as part of dairy checkoff program." March 1, 2018. https://www.dairyreporter.com/Article/2018/03/01/Pizza-Hut-adds-25-more-cheese-to-pan-pizzas-as-part-of-dairy-checkoff-program.

37   Michael Moss, Salt Sugar Fat: How the Food Giants Hooked Us, 2014. Random House Inc.

38   Katan, Martijn B. "Does industry sponsorship undermine the integrity of nutrition research?" *PLoS medicine* 4, no. 1 (2007): e6.

39   Keys, Ancel, Francisco Grande, and Joseph T. Anderson. "Bias and misrepresentation revisited: Perspective on saturated fat." The American journal of clinical nutrition 27, no. 2 (1974): 188-212. http://vorga.org/27-2-188.full.pdf.

40   Patty W Siri-Tarino, Qi Sun, Frank B Hu, Ronald M Krauss, "Meta-analysis of prospective cohort studies evaluating the association of saturated fat with cardiovascular disease," The American Journal of Clinical Nutrition, Volume 91, Issue 3, March 2010, Pages 535–546, https://doi.org/10.3945/ajcn.2009.27725.

41   Clarke, Robert, Chris Frost, Rory Collins, Paul Appleby, and Richard Peto. "Dietary lipids and blood cholesterol: quantitative meta-analysis of metabolic ward studies." Bmj 314, no. 7074 (1997): 112.

42   Anahad O'Connor. "Study Questions Fat and Heart Disease Link." The New York Times. March 17, 2014.

43   Walter Willett, Frank Sacks, and Meir Stampfer. "Dietary fat and heart disease study is seriously misleading." The Nutrition Source. Harvard T.H.Chan School of Public Health.

44   Julia Belluz. "Why it took the FDA nearly 40 years to ban trans fats." Vox. June 17, 2015.

45   Caitlin Dewey. "Artificial trans fats, widely linked to heart disease, are officially banned." The Washington Post. June 18, 2018.

46   Ibid.

47   Roberts, William Clifford. "It's the cholesterol, stupid!" American Journal of Cardiology 106, no. 9 (2010): 1364-1366.

48 Teo, Koon, Clara K. Chow, Mario Vaz, Sumathy Rangarajan, and Salim Yusuf. "The Prospective Urban Rural Epidemiology (PURE) study: examining the impact of societal influences on chronic noncommunicable diseases in low-, middle-, and high-income countries." American heart journal 158, no. 1 (2009): 1-7.

49 "PURE study makes headlines, but the conclusions are misleading," The Nutrition Source, Harvard T.H. Chan School of Public Health.

50 Miller, Victoria, Andrew Mente, Mahshid Dehghan, Sumathy Rangarajan, Xiaohe Zhang, Sumathi Swaminathan, Gilles Dagenais et al. "Fruit, vegetable, and legume intake, and cardiovascular disease and deaths in 18 countries (PURE): a prospective cohort study." The Lancet 390, no. 10107 (2017): 2037-2049.

51 Sacks, Frank M., Alice H. Lichtenstein, Jason HY Wu, Lawrence J. Appel, Mark A. Creager, Penny M. Kris-Etherton, Michael Miller et al. "Dietary fats and cardiovascular disease: a presidential advisory from the American Heart Association." Circulation 136, no. 3 (2017): e1-e23.

52 Steve White and Christopher Bucktin, "James Gandolfini's 'fried food feasty' before heart attack added up to 2,730 calories," The Mirror, September 10, 2013.

53 Abela, George S., Kusai Aziz, Ameeth Vedre, Dorothy R. Pathak, John D. Talbott, and Joyce DeJong. "Effect of cholesterol crystals on plaques and intima in arteries of patients with acute coronary and cerebrovascular syndromes." The American journal of cardiology 103, no. 7 (2009): 959-968.

54 Kloner, Robert A., W. Kenneth Poole, and Rebecca L. Perritt. "When throughout the year is coronary death most likely to occur? A 12-year population-based analysis of more than 220 000 cases." Circulation 100, no. 15 (1999): 1630-1634.

55 Seftel, Allen D., Peter Sun, and Ralph Swindle. "The prevalence of hypertension, hyperlipidemia, diabetes mellitus and depression in men with erectile dysfunction." The Journal of urology 171, no. 6 Part 1 (2004): 2341-2345.

56 Hanson AJ, Bayer-Carter JL, Green PS, et al. Effect of Apolipoprotein E Genotype and Diet on Apolipoprotein E Lipidation and Amyloid Peptides: Randomized Clinical Trial. JAMA Neurol. 2013;70(8):972-980. doi:10.1001/jamaneurol.2013.396.

57 Breteler, Monique MB. "Vascular risk factors for Alzheimer's disease: An epidemiologic perspective." Neurobiology of aging 21, no. 2 (2000): 153-160.

58 Spankovich, C., and C. G. Le Prell. "Healthy diets, healthy hearing: National health and nutrition examination survey, 1999–2002." International journal of audiology 52, no. 6 (2013): 369-376.

59 "The truth about fats: the good, the bad, and the in-between." August 2018. Harvard Health Publishing. https://www.health.harvard.edu/staying-healthy/the-truth-about-fats-bad-and-good.

60 Scott A, Zwerver J, Grewal N, *et al* Lipids, adiposity and tendinopathy: is there a mechanistic link? Critical review *British Journal of Sports Medicine* 2015; 49:984-988.

61 "Nonalcoholic fatty liver disease." Mayo Clinic. https://www.mayoclinic.org/diseases-conditions/nonalcoholic-fatty-liver-disease/symptoms-causes/syc-20354567.

62 Robb Wolf. "Episode 385—Dr. Shawn Baker—Carnivore Diet and Dr. Baker's Blood Work." Revolutionary Solutions to Modern Life. https://robbwolf.com/2018/03/13/episode-385-dr-shawn-baker-carnivore-diet-and-dr-bakers-blood-work/.

63 Keogh, Jennifer B., Jessica A. Grieger, Manny Noakes, and Peter M. Clifton. "Flow-mediated dilatation is impaired by a high-saturated fat diet but not by a high-carbohydrate diet." *Arteriosclerosis, thrombosis, and vascular biology* 25, no. 6 (2005): 1274-1279.

64 Vassallo, Ralph R., and Frank M. Stearns. "Lipemic plasma: a renaissance." Transfusion 51, no. 6 (2011): 1136-1139.

65 Esposito, Katherine, Miryam Ciotola, Ferdinando C. Sasso, Domenico Cozzolino, Franco Saccomanno, Roberta Assaloni, Antonio Ceriello, and Dario Giugliano. "Effect of a single high-fat meal on endothelial function in patients with the metabolic syndrome: role of tumor necrosis factor-α." Nutrition, metabolism and cardiovascular diseases 17, no. 4 (2007): 274-279.

66 Swank, Roy L. "Changes in blood of dogs and rabbits by high fat intake." American Journal of Physiology-Legacy Content 196, no. 3 (1959): 473-477.

67 Kennedy, Arion, Kristina Martinez, Chia-Chi Chuang, Kathy LaPoint, and Michael McIntosh. "Saturated fatty acid-mediated inflammation and insulin resistance in adipose tissue: mechanisms of action and implications." *The Journal of nutrition* 139, no. 1 (2008): 1-4.

68 Connor, William E., John C. Hoak, and Emory D. Warner. "Massive thrombosis produced by fatty acid infusion." *The Journal of clinical investigation* 42, no. 6 (1963): 860-866.

69 Vogel, Robert A., Mary C. Corretti, and Gary D. Plotnick. "Effect of a single high-fat meal on endothelial function in healthy subjects." *The American journal of cardiology* 79, no. 3 (1997): 350-354.

70 Marchesi, Simona, Graziana Lupattelli, Giuseppe Schillaci, Matteo Pirro, Donatella Siepi, Anna Rita Roscini, Leonella Pasqualini, and Elmo Mannarino. "Impaired flow-mediated vasoactivity during post-prandial phase in young healthy men." *Atherosclerosis* 153, no. 2 (2000): 397-402.

71 Quintanilha, Bruna Jardim, Ludmila Rodrigues Pinto Ferreira, Frederico Moraes Ferreira, Edécio Cunha Neto, Geni Rodrigues Sampaio, and Marcelo Macedo Rogero. "Circulating plasma microRNAs dysregulation and metabolic endotoxemia induced by a high-fat high-saturated diet."*Clinical Nutrition* (2019).

72 Grundy, Scott M., Neil J. Stone, Alison L. Bailey, Craig Beam, Kim K. Birtcher, Roger S. Blumenthal, Lynne T. Braun et al. "2018 AHA/ACC/AACVPR/ AAPA/ABC/ACPM/ADA/AGS/APhA/ASPC/NLA/PCNA guideline on the management of blood cholesterol: a report of the American College of Cardiology/American Heart Association Task Force on Clinical Practice Guidelines." *Journal of the American College of Cardiology* (2018): 25709.

73 O'Keefe, James H., Loren Cordain, William H. Harris, Richard M. Moe, and Robert Vogel. "Optimal low-density lipoprotein is 50 to 70 mg/dl: lower is better and physiologically normal." Journal of the American College of Cardiology 43, no. 11 (2004): 2142-2146.

74 Rosinger, Asher, Margaret D. Carroll, David Lacher, and Cynthia Ogden. "Trends in total cholesterol, triglycerides, and low-density lipoprotein in US adults, 1999-2014." *JAMA cardiology* 2, no. 3 (2017): 339-341.

75 Kuklina EV, Carroll MD, Shaw KM, Hirsch R. "Trends in high LDL cholesterol, cholesterol-lowering medication use, and dietary saturated-fat intake: United States," 1976-2010. NCHS data brief, no 117. Hyattsville, MD: National Center for Health Statistics. 2013.

76 Kuklina EV, Carroll MD, Shaw KM, Hirsch R. "Trends in high LDL cholesterol, cholesterol-lowering medication use, and dietary saturated-fat intake: United States," 1976-2010. NCHS data brief, no 117. Hyattsville, MD: National Center for Health Statistics. 2013.

77 Brian A. Ference, Henry N. Ginsberg, Ian Graham, Kausik K. Ray, Chris J. Packard, Eric Bruckert, Robert A. Hegele, Ronald M. Krauss, Frederick J. Raal, Heribert Schunkert, Gerald F. Watts, Jan Borén, Sergio Fazio, Jay D. Horton, Luis Masana, Stephen J. Nicholls, Børge. Nordestgaard, Bart van de Sluis, Marja-Riitta Taskinen, Lale Tokgözoğlu, Ulf Landmesser, Ulrich Laufs, Olov Wiklund, Jane K. Stock, M. John Chapman, Alberico L. Catapano, "Low-density lipoproteins cause atherosclerotic cardiovascular disease. 1. Evidence from genetic, epidemiologic, and clinical studies. A consensus statement from the European Atherosclerosis Society Consensus Panel," *European Heart Journal*, Volume 38, Issue 32, 21 August 2017, Pages 2459-2472, https://doi. org/10.1093/eurheartj/ehx144.

78 The International Network of Cholesterol Skeptics, https://www.thincs.org/.

79 Ference, Brian A., Henry N. Ginsberg, Ian Graham, Kausik K. Ray, Chris J. Packard, Eric Bruckert, Robert A. Hegele et al. "Low-density lipoproteins cause atherosclerotic cardiovascular disease. 1. Evidence from genetic, epidemiologic, and clinical studies. A consensus statement from the European Atherosclerosis Society Consensus Panel." European heart journal 38, no. 32 (2017): 2459-2472.

80 https://twitter.com/mvholmes/status/1114537166145769473?s=20.

81 Heron, Melonie. "Deaths: Leading Causes for 2016." National Vital Statistics Reports, No 6, Vol. 67.

82 Martin S.S., Blumenthal R.S., Miller M. "LDL Cholesterol: The Lower the Better." 2012. Medical Clinics of North America, 96 (1), pp. 13-26.

83 Roberts, William Clifford. "It's the cholesterol, stupid!" American Journal of Cardiology 106, no. 9 (2010): 1364-1366.

84 Bibbins-Domingo, Kirsten, David C. Grossman, Susan J. Curry, Karina W. Davidson, John W. Epling, Francisco AR García, Matthew W. Gillman et al. "Statin use for the primary prevention of cardiovascular disease in adults: US Preventive Services Task Force recommendation statement." Jama 316, no. 19 (2016): 1997-2007.

85 Sara G. Miller, "Why Americans' Cholesterol Levels Are Improving." Live Science. November 30, 2016. https://www.livescience.com/57020-cholesterol-level-trends.html.

86 Austin, Melissa A., Carolyn M. Hutter, Ron L. Zimmern, and Steve E. Humphries. "Genetic causes of monogenic heterozygous familial hypercholesterolemia: a HuGE prevalence review." American journal of epidemiology 160, no. 5 (2004): 407-420.

87 Ibid.

88 Curb, Jess D., and Kazunori Kodama. "The Ni-Hon-San Study." Journal of Epidemiology 6, no. 4sup (1996): 197-201.

89 Connor, William E., Maria Teresa Cerqueira, Rodney W. Connor, Robert B. Wallace, M. René Malinow, and H. Richard Casdorph. "The plasma lipids, lipoproteins, and diet of the Tarahumara Indians of Mexico." The American journal of clinical nutrition 31, no. 7 (1978): 1131-1142.

90 Khera, Amit V., Connor A. Emdin, Isabel Drake, Pradeep Natarajan, Alexander G. Bick, Nancy R. Cook, Daniel I. Chasman et al. "Genetic risk, adherence to a healthy lifestyle, and coronary disease." *New England Journal of Medicine* 375, no. 24 (2016): 2349-2358.

91 Nordestgaard, Børge G., M. John Chapman, Steve E. Humphries, Henry N. Ginsberg, Luis Masana, Olivier S. Descamps, Olov Wiklund et al. "Familial hypercholesterolaemia is underdiagnosed and undertreated in the general population: guidance for clinicians to prevent coronary heart disease: consensus statement of the European Atherosclerosis Society." *European heart journal* 34, no. 45 (2013): 3478-3490.

92 Freedman, David S., William H. Dietz, Sathanur R. Srinivasan, and Gerald S. Berenson. "The relation of overweight to cardiovascular risk factors among children and adolescents: the Bogalusa Heart Study." Pediatrics 103, no. 6 (1999): 1175-1182.

93 Kempner, W. (1948). "Treatment of hypertensive vascular disease with rice diet." *The American journal of medicine*, 4(4), 545-577.

94 Satija, Ambika, Shilpa N. Bhupathiraju, Eric B. Rimm, Donna Spiegelman, Stephanie E. Chiuve, Lea Borgi, Walter C. Willett, JoAnn E. Manson, Qi Sun, and Frank B. Hu. "Plant-based dietary patterns and incidence of type 2 diabetes in US men and women: results from three prospective cohort studies." *PLoS medicine* 13, no. 6 (2016): e1002039.

95 Clarke, Robert, Chris Frost, Rory Collins, Paul Appleby, and Richard Peto. "Dietary lipids and blood cholesterol: quantitative meta-analysis of metabolic ward studies." Bmj 314, no. 7074 (1997): 112.

96 Keys, A. and Parlin, R. W. 1966. "Serum cholesterol response to changes in dietary lipids." *The American journal of clinical nutrition*, 19(3), 175-181.

97 Mozaffarian, D., Benjamin, E. J., Go, A. S., Arnett, D. K., Blaha, M. J., Cushman, M., ...& Howard, V. J. (2016). "Heart disease and stroke statistics-2016 update a report from the American Heart Association." Circulation, 133(4), e38-e48.

98 https://www.cargill.com/about/financial-information.

99 https://www.marketwatch.com/investing/stock/tsn/financials.

100 http://diabetes.diabetesjournals.org/content/67/1/3.

101 Yuhara, H., Steinmaus, C., Cohen, S. E., Corley, D. A., Tei, Y., & Buffler, P. A. (2011). "Is diabetes mellitus an independent risk factor for colon cancer and rectal cancer?" *The American journal of gastroenterology*, 106(11), 1911.

102 Lean, Michael EJ, Wilma S. Leslie, Alison C. Barnes, Naomi Brosnahan, George Thom, Louise McCombie, Carl Peters et al. "Primary care-led weight management for remission of type 2 diabetes (DiRECT): an open-label, cluster-randomised trial." The Lancet 391, no. 10120 (2018): 541-551.

103 Paschos, P., & Paletas, K. (2009). "Non alcoholic fatty liver disease and metabolic syndrome." Hippokratia, 13(1), 9.

104 Luukkonen, Panu K., Sanja Sädevirta, You Zhou, Brandon Kayser, Ashfaq Ali, Linda Ahonen, Susanna Lallukka et al. "Saturated fat is more metabolically harmful for the human liver than unsaturated fat or simple sugars." Diabetes care 41, no. 8 (2018): 1732-1739.

105 Winzell, M. S., & Ahrén, B. (2004). "The high-fat diet-fed mouse: a model for studying mechanisms and treatment of impaired glucose tolerance and type 2 diabetes." Diabetes, 53(suppl 3), S215-S219.

106 Robertson, M. D., Kim G. Jackson, B. A. Fielding, Christine M. Williams, and K. N. Frayn. "Acute effects of meal fatty acid composition on insulin sensitivity in healthy post-menopausal women." British journal of nutrition 88, no. 6 (2002): 635-640.

107 Unger, R. H., & Zhou, Y. T. (2001). Lipotoxicity of beta-cells in obesity and in other causes of fatty acid spillover. Diabetes, 50(suppl 1), S118.

108 Tonstad, Serena, K. Stewart, K. Oda, M. Batech, R. P. Herring, and G. E. Fraser. "Vegetarian diets and incidence of diabetes in the Adventist Health Study-2." Nutrition, Metabolism and Cardiovascular Diseases 23, no. 4 (2013): 292-299.

109 Goff, Louise M., Jimmy D. Bell, P-W. So, Anne Dornhorst, and G. S. Frost. "Veganism and its relationship with insulin resistance and intramyocellular lipid." European journal of clinical nutrition 59, no. 2 (2005): 291.

110 Anderson, James W., and Kyleen Ward. "High-carbohydrate, high-fiber diets for insulin-treated men with diabetes mellitus." The American journal of clinical nutrition 32, no. 11 (1979): 2312-2321.

111 Chiu, Tina HT, Hui-Ya Huang, Yen-Feng Chiu, Wen-Harn Pan, Hui-Yi Kao, Jason PC Chiu, Ming-Nan Lin, and Chin-Lon Lin. "Taiwanese vegetarians and omnivores: dietary composition, prevalence of diabetes and IFG." PLoS One 9, no. 2 (2014): e88547.

112 Guasch-Ferré, Marta, Nerea Becerra-Tomas, Miguel Ruiz-Canela, Dolores Corella, Helmut Schröder, Ramon Estruch, Emilio Ros et al. "Total and subtypes of dietary fat intake and risk of type 2 diabetes mellitus in the Prevención con Dieta Mediterránea (PREDIMED) study." The American journal of clinical nutrition 105, no. 3 (2017): 723-735.

113 Diabetes UK. January 23, 2017. "Eating saturated fat has immediate effect on your liver." https://www.diabetes.org.uk/research/research-round-up/eating-saturated-fat-has-immediate-effect-on-your-liver.

114 Sweency, J. Shirley. "Dietary factors that influence the dextrose tolerance test: a preliminary study." Archives of Internal Medicine 40, no. 6 (1927): 818-830.

115 Chapman, Carleton B., Thomas Gibbons, and Austin Henschel. "The effect of the rice-fruit diet on the composition of the body." New England Journal of Medicine 243, no. 23 (1950): 899-905.

116 Joslin, E. P. (1930). Arteriosclerosis in diabetes. *Annals of Internal Medicine*, 4(1), 54-66.

117 Wan, Yi, Fenglei Wang, Jinhong Yuan, and Duo Li. "Optimal dietary macronutrient distribution in China (ODMDC): A randomised controlled-feeding trial protocol." *Asia Pacific journal of clinical nutrition* 26, no. 5 (2017): 972.

118 Luukkonen, Panu K., Sanja Sädevirta, You Zhou, Brandon Kayser, Ashfaq Ali, Linda Ahonen, Susanna Lallukka et al. "Saturated fat is more metabolically harmful for the human liver than unsaturated fat or simple sugars." Diabetes care 41, no. 8 (2018): 1732-1739.

119 Stefan, Norbert, and Hans-Ulrich Häring. "The metabolically benign and malignant fatty liver." Diabetes 60, no. 8 (2011).

120 McKenzie, Amy L., Sarah J. Hallberg, Brent C. Creighton, Brittanie M. Volk, Theresa M. Link, Marcy K. Abner, Roberta M. Glon, James P. McCarter, Jeff S. Volek, and Stephen D. Phinney. "A novel intervention including individualized nutritional recommendations reduces hemoglobin A1c level, medication use, and weight in type 2 diabetes." *JMIR diabetes* 2, no. 1 (2017): e5.

121 McKenzie, Amy L., Sarah J. Hallberg, Brent C. Creighton, Brittanie M. Volk, Theresa M. Link, Marcy K. Abner, Roberta M. Glon, James P. McCarter, Jeff S. Volek, and Stephen D. Phinney. "A novel intervention including individualized nutritional recommendations reduces hemoglobin A1c level, medication use, and weight in type 2 diabetes." JMIR diabetes2, no. 1 (2017): e5.

122 Bhanpuri, Nasir H., Sarah J. Hallberg, Paul T. Williams, Amy L. McKenzie, Kevin D. Ballard, Wayne W. Campbell, James P. McCarter, Stephen D. Phinney, and Jeff S. Volek. "Cardiovascular disease risk factor responses to a type 2 diabetes care model including nutritional ketosis induced by sustained carbohydrate restriction at 1 year: an open label, non-randomized, controlled study." *Cardiovascular diabetology* 17, no. 1 (2018): 56.

123 McKenzie, Amy L., Sarah J. Hallberg, Brent C. Creighton, Brittanie M. Volk, Theresa M. Link, Marcy K. Abner, Roberta M. Glon, James P. McCarter, Jeff S. Volek, and Stephen D. Phinney. "A novel intervention including individualized nutritional recommendations reduces hemoglobin A1c level, medication use, and weight in type 2 diabetes." *JMIR diabetes2*, no. 1 (2017): e5.

124 Dr. Joel Kahn. 2017. "The Skeleton in The Ketogenic Diet Closet." https://medium.com/thrive-global/the-skeleton-in-the-ketogenic-diet-closet-what-virta-health-mark-sisson-joseph-mercola-and-704fad8bffd7.

125 Li, Shanshan, Alan Flint, Jennifer K. Pai, John P. Forman, Frank B. Hu, Walter C. Willett, Kathryn M. Rexrode, Kenneth J. Mukamal, and Eric B. Rimm. "Low carbohydrate diet from plant or animal sources and mortality among myocardial infarction survivors." *Journal of the American Heart Association* 3, no. 5 (2014): e001169.

126 Noto, Hiroshi, Atsushi Goto, Tetsuro Tsujimoto, and Mitsuhiko Noda. "Low-carbohydrate diets and all-cause mortality: a systematic review and meta-analysis of observational studies." *PloS one* 8, no. 1 (2013): e55030.

127 Hallberg, Sarah J., Amy L. McKenzie, Paul T. Williams, Nasir H. Bhanpuri, Anne L. Peters, Wayne W. Campbell, Tamara L. Hazbun et al. "Effectiveness and safety of a novel care model for the management of type 2 diabetes at 1 year: an open-label, non-randomized, controlled study." Diabetes Therapy 9, no. 2 (2018): 583 612.

128 Guasch-Ferré, Marta, Nerea Becerra-Tomas, Miguel Ruiz-Canela, Dolores Corella, Helmut Schröder, Ramon Estruch, Emilio Ros et al. "Total and subtypes of dietary fat intake and risk of type 2 diabetes mellitus in the Prevención con Dieta Mediterránea (PREDIMED) study." *The American journal of clinical nutrition* 105, no. 3 (2017): 723-735.

129 InterAct Consortium. "Association between dietary meat consumption and incident type 2 diabetes: the EPIC-InterAct study." *Diabetologia* 56, no. 1 (2013): 47-59.

130 Brad Plumer. "How Much of the world's cropland is actually used to grow food?" https://www.vox.com/2014/8/21/6053187/cropland-map-food-fuel-animal-feed.

131 Anup Shah. "Diverting resources to environmentally destructive uses." http://www.globalissues.org/article/240/beef.

132 "Why Aren't We Eating More Insects?" September 2018. The New York Times Style Magazine. https://www.nytimes.com/2018/09/07/t-magazine/eating-bugs-food-restaurant.html.

133 Chaurasia, Bhagirath, Vincent Andre Kaddai, Graeme Iain Lancaster, Darren C. Henstridge, Sandhya Sriram, Dwight Lark Anolin Galam, Venkatesh Gopalan et al. "Adipocyte ceramides regulate subcutaneous adipose browning, inflammation, and metabolism." Cell metabolism 24, no. 6 (2016): 820-834.

134 Chaurasia, Bhagirath, Vincent Andre Kaddai, Graeme Iain Lancaster, Darren C. Henstridge, Sandhya Sriram, Dwight Lark Anolin Galam, Venkatesh Gopalan et al. "Adipocyte ceramides regulate subcutaneous adipose browning, inflammation, and metabolism." *Cell metabolism* 24, no. 6 (2016): 820-834.

135 Chaurasia, Bhagirath, and Scott A. Summers. "Ceramides–lipotoxic inducers of metabolic disorders." Trends in Endocrinology & Metabolism 26, no. 10 (2015): 538-550.

136 "Controlling ceramides could help treat heart disease." March 2018. https://www.sbpdiscovery.org/press/controlling-ceramides-could-help-treat-heart-disease.

137 Lin, Guang, Pei-Tseng Lee, Kuchuan Chen, Dongxue Mao, Kai Li Tan, Zhongyuan Zuo, Wen-Wen Lin, Liping Wang, and Hugo J. Bellen. "Phospholipase PLA2G6, a parkinsonism-associated gene, affects Vps26 and Vps35, retromer function, and ceramide levels, similar to α-synuclein gain." *Cell metabolism* 28, no. 4 (2018): 605-618.

138 Swank, Roy L. "Treatment of multiple sclerosis with low-fat diet." AMA Archives of Neurology & Psychiatry 69, no. 1 (1953): 91-103.

139 Kurz, Jennifer, Robert Brunkhorst, Christian Foerch, Leonard Blum, Marina Henke, Laureen Gabriel, Thomas Ulshöfer et al. "The relevance of ceramides and their synthesizing enzymes for multiple sclerosis." Clinical Science 132, no. 17 (2018): 1963-1976.

140 Moro, Kazuki, Tsutomu Kawaguchi, Junko Tsuchida, Emmanuel Gabriel, Qianya Qi, Li Yan, Toshifumi Wakai, Kazuaki Takabe, and Masayuki Nagahashi. "Ceramide species are elevated in human breast cancer and are associated with less aggressiveness." *Oncotarget* 9, no. 28 (2018): 19874.

141 Lopez, Ximena, Allison B. Goldfine, William L. Holland, Ruth Gordillo, and Philipp E. Scherer. "Plasma ceramides are elevated in female children and adolescents with type 2 diabetes." *Journal of Pediatric Endocrinology and Metabolism* 26, no. 9-10 (2013): 995-998.

142 Haus, Jacob M., Sangeeta R. Kashyap, Takhar Kasumov, Renliang Zhang, Karen R. Kelly, Ralph A. DeFronzo, and John P. Kirwan. "Plasma ceramides are elevated in obese subjects with type 2 diabetes and correlate with the severity of insulin resistance." Diabetes 58, no. 2 (2009): 337-343.

143 Davis, A. N., J. E. Rico, W. A. Myers, M. E. Coleman, M. E. Clapham, N. J. Haughey, and J. W. McFadden. "Circulating low-density lipoprotein ceramide concentrations increase in Holstein dairy cows transitioning from gestation to lactation." Journal of dairy science (2019).

144 Caroprese, Mariangela, A. Marzano, G. Entrican, S. Wattegedera, Marzia Albenzio, and Agostino Sevi. "Immune response of cows fed polyunsaturated fatty acids under high ambient temperatures." *Journal of dairy science* 92, no. 6 (2009): 2796-2803.

145 Diop, Soda Balla, Jumana Bisharat-Kernizan, Ryan Tyge Birse, Sean Oldham, Karen Ocorr, and Rolf Bodmer. "PGC-1/spargel counteracts high-fat-diet-induced obesity and cardiac lipotoxicity downstream of TOR and brummer ATGL lipase." *Cell reports* 10, no. 9 (2015): 1572-1584.

146 Mary Caffrey. 2017. "Ceramides Can Predict Who Will Develop Heart Disease, Study Finds." https://www.ajmc.com/conferences/acc-2017/ceramides-can-predict-who-will-develop-heart-disease-study-finds.

147 Chaurasia, Bhagirath, and Scott A. Summers. "Ceramides–lipotoxic inducers of metabolic disorders." Trends in Endocrinology & Metabolism 26, no. 10 (2015): 538-550.

148 Holland, William L., Benjamin T. Bikman, Li-Ping Wang, Guan Yuguang, Katherine M. Sargent, Sarada Bulchand, Trina A. Knotts et al. "Lipid-induced insulin resistance mediated by the proinflammatory receptor TLR4 requires saturated fatty acid–induced ceramide biosynthesis in mice." *The Journal of clinical investigation* 121, no. 5 (2011): 1858-1870.

149 Chavez, Jose Antonio, Trina A. Knotts, Li-Ping Wang, Guibin Li, Rick T. Dobrowsky, Gregory L. Florant, and Scott A. Summers. "A role for ceramide, but not diacylglycerol, in the antagonism of insulin signal transduction by saturated fatty acids." *Journal of Biological Chemistry* 278, no. 12 (2003): 10297-10303.

150 Pagadala, Mangesh, Takhar Kasumov, Arthur J. McCullough, Nizar N. Zein, and John P. Kirwan. "Role of ceramides in nonalcoholic fatty liver disease." Trends in Endocrinology & Metabolism 23, no. 8 (2012): 365-371.

151 Alzheimer's disease is not synonymous with dementia. Dementia is a variety of medical conditions and illnesses that impair a person's cognitive health, and Alzheimer's is one type of dementia. Senile dementia is the mental deterioration associated with age, and there are two major types: Alzheimer's-type dementia, which is due to general atrophy, and vascular dementia, which results from damage to the vessels supplying blood to the brain. There are also Lewy body dementia, Frontotemporal dementia, and mixed dementia, which is when a patient has Alzheimer's disease, vascular dementia, and Lewy body dementia.

152 Roher, Alex E., Chera Esh, Tyler A. Kokjohn, Walter Kalback, Dean C. Luehrs, James D. Seward, Lucia I. Sue, and Thomas G. Beach. "Circle of Willis atherosclerosis is a risk factor for sporadic Alzheimer's disease." Arteriosclerosis, Thrombosis, and Vascular Biology 23, no. 11 (2003): 2055-2062.

153 Breteler, Monique MB. "Vascular risk factors for Alzheimer's disease: An epidemiologic perspective." Neurobiology of aging 21, no. 2 (2000): 153-160.

154 Dede, Didem Sener, Bunyamin Yavuz, Burcu Balam Yavuz, Mustafa Cankurtaran, Meltem Halil, Zekeriya Ulger, Eylem Sahin Cankurtaran, Kudret Aytemir, Giray Kabakci, and Servet Ariogul. "Assessment of endothelial function in Alzheimer's disease: is Alzheimer's disease a vascular disease?" Journal of the American Geriatrics Society 55, no. 10 (2007): 1613-1617.

155 Gottesman, Rebecca F., Andrea LC Schneider, Yun Zhou, Josef Coresh, Edward Green, Naresh Gupta, David S. Knopman et al. "Association between midlife vascular risk factors and estimated brain amyloid deposition." JAMA 317, no. 14 (2017): 1443-1450.

156 Hofman, Albert, Alewijn Ott, Monique MB Breteler, Michiel L. Bots, Arjen JC Slooter, Frans van Harskamp, Cornelia N. van Duijn, Christine Van Broeckhoven, and Diederick E. Grobbee. "Atherosclerosis, apolipoprotein E, and prevalence of dementia and Alzheimer's disease in the Rotterdam Study." The Lancet 349, no. 9046 (1997): 151-154.

157 Dede, Didem Sener, Bunyamin Yavuz, Burcu Balam Yavuz, Mustafa Cankurtaran, Meltem Halil, Zekeriya Ulger, Eylem Sahin Cankurtaran, Kudret Aytemir, Giray Kabakci, and Servet Ariogul. "Assessment of endothelial function in Alzheimer's disease: is Alzheimer's disease a vascular disease?" Journal of the American Geriatrics Society 55, no. 10 (2007): 1613-1617.

158 Peter Kevern. 2017. "Why are we so afraid of dementia?" The Conversation. https://theconversation.com/why-are-we-so-afraid-of-dementia-83175.

159 Alzheimer's Association. 2018. Facts and Figures on Alzheimer's. https://www.alz.org/alzheimers-dementia/facts-figures.

160 Alisha Rouse. 2015. "Rise of patients in 40s suffering from dementia: Researchers warn of a 'silent epidemic' of early onset of the disease." The Daily Mail. https://www.dailymail.co.uk/news/article-3186583/Rise-patients-40s-suffering-dementia-Researchers-warn-silent-epidemic-early-onset-disease.html.

161 Hanson, Angela J., Jennifer L. Bayer-Carter, Pattie S. Green, Thomas J. Montine, Charles W. Wilkinson, Laura D. Baker, G. Stennis Watson et al. "Effect of apolipoprotein E genotype and diet on apolipoprotein E lipidation and amyloid peptides: randomized clinical trial." JAMA neurology 70, no. 8 (2013): 972-980.

162 Dennis Thompson. "Saturated Fat May Make the Brain Vulnerable to Alzheimer's." HealthDay, June, 17, 2013. https://consumer.healthday.com/senior-citizen-information-31/age-health-news-7/saturated-fat-may-make-the-brain-vulnerable-to-alzheimer-s-677450.html.

163 Puglielli, Luigi, Rudolph E. Tanzi, and Dora M. Kovacs. "Alzheimer's disease: the cholesterol connection." Nature neuroscience 6, no. 4 (2003): 345.

164 Morris, M. C. "The role of nutrition in Alzheimer's disease: epidemiological evidence." European Journal of Neurology 16 (2009): 1-7.

165 Morris, Martha Clare, Denis A. Evans, Julia L. Bienias, Christine C. Tangney, David A. Bennett, Neelum Aggarwal, Julie Schneider, and Robert S. Wilson. "Dietary fats and the risk of incident Alzheimer disease." Archives of neurology 60, no. 2 (2003): 194-200.

166 Jick, H. Z. G. L., Gwen L. Zornberg, Susan S. Jick, Sudha Seshadri, and David A. Drachman. "Statins and the risk of dementia." The Lancet 356, no. 9242 (2000): 1627-1631.

167 Morris, Martha Clare, Denis A. Evans, Julia L. Bienias, Christine C. Tangney, David A. Bennett, Neelum Aggarwal, Julie Schneider, and Robert S. Wilson. "Dietary fats and the risk of incident Alzheimer disease." Archives of neurology 60, no. 2 (2003): 194-200.

168 Engelhart, M. J., M. I. Geerlings, A. Ruitenberg, J. C. Van Swieten, A. Hofman, J. C. M. Witteman, and M. M. B. Breteler. "Diet and risk of dementia: Does fat matter?: The Rotterdam Study." Neurology 59, no. 12 (2002): 1915-1921.

169 Cervantes, Breana, and Lynn Ulatowski. "Vitamin E and Alzheimer's disease—Is it time for personalized medicine?" Antioxidants 6, no. 3 (2017): 45.

170 Giem, Paul, W. Lawrence Beeson, and Gary E. Fraser. "The incidence of dementia and intake of animal products: preliminary findings from the Adventist Health Study." Neuroepidemiology 12, no. 1 (1993): 28-36.

171 Alzheimer, A. "Über eine eigenartige Erkrankung der Hirnrinde." Allgemeine Zeitschrift fur Psychiatrie under Psychisch-Gerichtliche Medizin." (1907): 146-8.

172 Armstrong, Mark L., Emory D. Warner, and William E. Connor. "Regression of coronary atheromatosis in rhesus monkeys." Circulation research 27, no. 1 (1970): 59-67.

173 Eggen, Douglas A., Jack P. Strong, William P. Newman, Gray T. Malcom, and Carlos Restrepo. "Regression of experimental atherosclerotic lesions in rhesus monkeys consuming a high saturated fat diet." Arteriosclerosis: An Official Journal of the American Heart Association, Inc. 7, no. 2 (1987): 125-134.

174 Billings, James H., Larry W. Scherwitz, Rick Sullivan, Stephen Sparler, and Dean M. Ornish. "The Lifestyle Heart Trial: Comprehensive treatment and group support therapy." (1996).

175 Hubbard, Jeffrey D., Stephen Inkeles, and R. James Barnard. "Nathan Pritikin's heart." The New England journal of medicine 313, no. 1 (1985): 52-52.

176 Dan Buettner. 2015. *The Blue Zones Solution: Eating and Living Like the World's Healthiest People.* National Geographic Books. 2015.

177 Keys, Ancel, Alessandro Menotti, Christ Aravanis, Henry Blackburn, Bozidar S. Djordević, Ratko Buzina, A. S. Dontas et al. "The seven countries study: 2,289 deaths in 15 years." Preventive medicine 13, no. 2 (1984): 141-154.

178 The Seven Countries Study. Average saturated fat intake and CHD mortality rates. https://www.sevencountriesstudy.com/ average-saturated-fat-intake-and-coronary-heart-disease-rates-in-the-16-cohorts/#prettyPhoto[fancy_img_group_171]/0/.

179 The Seven Countries Study. Serum cholesterol and coronary heart disease. https://www.helsinki.fi/en/news/nordic-welfare/ north-karelia-project-an-unrepeatable-success-story-in-public-health.

180 Dan Buettner. 2015. *The Blue Zones Solution: Eating and Living Like the World's Healthiest People.* National Geographic Books. 2015.

181 Puska, Pekka. "Successful prevention of non-communicable diseases: 25 year experiences with North Karelia Project in Finland." Public Health Medicine 4, no. 1 (2002): 5-7.

182 Johannes Kananen. *North Karelia Project—An unrepeatable success story in public health.* Nordic Health News. University of Helsinki. https://www.helsinki.fi/en/news/nordic-welfare/ north-karelia-project-an-unrepeatable-success-story-in-public-health.

183 Hindhede, Mikkel. "The effect of food restriction during war on mortality in Copenhagen." *Journal of the American Medical Association* 74, no. 6 (1920): 381-382.

184 The Norwegian University of Science and Technology (NTNU). "Heart and cardiovascular disease deaths drop dramatically in Norway." ScienceDaily. www.sciencedaily.com/releases/2011/03/110318160927.htm (accessed April 21, 2019).

185 Stewart Ross. "Rationing: Could the WW2 diet make you healthier?" British Broadcasting Corporation. http://www.bbc.co.uk/guides/zqftn39.

186 Young, F.G., and K.C. Richardson. "Discussion on the cause of diabetes." *Proceedings of the Royal Society of Medicine* vol. 42,5 (1949): 321-30.

187 Mark Easton. "The mystery of the 'golden cohort.'" British Broadcasting Corporation. https://www.bbc.com/news/uk-15024436.

188 Franco, Manuel, Usama Bilal, Pedro Orduñez, Mikhail Benet, Alain Morejón, Benjamín Caballero, Joan F. Kennelly, and Richard S. Cooper. "Population-wide weight loss and regain in relation to diabetes burden and cardiovascular mortality in Cuba 1980-2010: repeated cross sectional surveys and ecological comparison of secular trends." *Bmj* 346 (2013): f1515.

189 Richard Schiffman. "How Cubans' Health Improved When Their Economy Collapsed." The Atlantic. April 18, 2013. https://www.theatlantic.com/health/archive/2013/04/how-cubans-health-improved-when-their-economy-collapsed/275080/.

190 Rodríguez-Ojea, Arturo, Santa Jiménez, Antonio Berdasco, and Mercedes Esquivel. "The nutrition transition in Cuba in the nineties: an overview." *Public Health Nutrition* 5, no. 1a (2002): 129-133.

191 Franco, Manuel, Usama Bilal, Pedro Orduñez, Mikhail Benet, Alain Morejón, Benjamín Caballero, Joan F. Kennelly, and Richard S. Cooper. "Population-wide weight loss and regain in relation to diabetes burden and cardiovascular mortality in Cuba 1980-2010: repeated cross sectional surveys and ecological comparison of secular trends." *Bmj* 346 (2013): f1515.

192 Najjar, Rami S., Carolyn E. Moore, and Baxter D. Montgomery. "A defined, plant-based diet utilized in an outpatient cardiovascular clinic effectively treats hypercholesterolemia and hypertension and reduces medications." *Clinical cardiology* 41, no. 3 (2018): 307-313.

193 Najjar, Rami S., Carolyn E. Moore, and Baxter D. Montgomery. "Consumption of a defined, plant-based diet reduces lipoprotein (a), inflammation, and other atherogenic lipoproteins and particles within 4 weeks." *Clinical cardiology* 41, no. 8 (2018): 1062-1068.

194 Arden Dier. "Canadian kale salad offers more calories, salt, and fat: CBC." Canadian Broadcasting Corporation. https://www.newser.com/story/220108/mcdonalds-salad-worse-than-a-double-big-mac.html.

195 Alice Philipson. "Italians lose appetite for healthy Mediterranean diet." The London Telegraph. December 2015. https://www.telegraph.co.uk/news/worldnews/europe/italy/12072005/Italians-lose-appetite-for-healthy-Mediterranean-diet.html.

196 Knowler, William C., Elizabeth Barrett-Connor, Sarah E. Fowler, Richard F. Hamman, John M. Lachin, Elizabeth A. Walker, and David M. Nathan. "Reduction in the incidence of type 2 diabetes with lifestyle intervention or metformin." *The New England journal of medicine* 346, no. 6 (2002): 393-403.

197 "University disavows chocolate milk, concussions study." CBS News. April 1, 2016. https://www.cbsnews.com/news/university-disavows-chocolate-milk-concussions-study/.

198 Daniel, C. R., Cross, A. J., Koebnick, C., & Sinha, R. (2010). Trends in meat consumption in the USA. *Public health nutrition*, 14(4), 575–583. doi:10.1017/S1368980010002077.

199 Ganmaa, D., P. Y. Wang, L. Q. Qin, K. Hoshi, and A. Sato. "Is milk responsible for male reproductive disorders?" *Medical hypotheses* 57, no. 4 (2001): 510-514.

200 Jouan, Pierre-Nicolas, Yves Pouliot, Sylvie F. Gauthier, and Jean-Paul Laforest. "Hormones in bovine milk and milk products: A survey." *International Dairy Journal* 16, no. 11 (2006): 1408-1414.

201 Afeiche, M., P. L. Williams, J. Mendiola, A. J. Gaskins, N. Jørgensen, S. H. Swan, and J. E. Chavarro. "Dairy food intake in relation to semen quality and reproductive hormone levels among physically active young men." *Human reproduction* 28, no. 8 (2013): 2265-2275.0.

202 Baldini, Marta, Francesca Pasqui, Alessandra Bordoni, and Magda Maranesi. "Is the Mediterranean lifestyle still a reality? Evaluation of food consumption and energy expenditure in Italian and Spanish university students." *Public health nutrition* 12, no. 2 (2009): 148-155.

203 Kelsey Casselbury. "The Average Fat Intake in SAD." November 19, 2018. SFGate. https://healthyeating.sfgate.com/average-fat-intake-sad-11370.html.

204 Andrew Jacobs. "How Chummy Are Junk Food Giants and China's Health Officials? They Share Offices." The New York Times. January 9, 2019. https://www.nytimes.com/2019/01/09/health/obesity-china-coke.html?rref=collection%2Fseriescollection%2Fobesity-epidemic&action=click&contentCollection=health&region=stream&module=stream_unit&version=latest&contentPlacement=1&pgtype=collection.

205 Greenhalgh, Susan. "Soda industry influence on obesity science and policy in China." *Journal of public health policy* 40, no. 1 (2019): 5-16.

206 Greenhalgh, Susan. "Making China safe for Coke: how Coca-Cola shaped obesity science and policy in China." *Bmj* 364 (2019): k5050.

207 Anahad O'Connor. "Coca-Cola Funds Scientists Who Shift Blame for Obesity Away From Bad Diets." New York Times. August 9, 2015. https://well.blogs.nytimes.com/2015/08/09/coca-cola-funds-scientists-who-shift-blame-for-obesity-away-from-bad-diets/.

208 "Different Dietary Fat, Different risk of Mortality." The Nutrition Source. Harvard T./H. Chan School of Public Health. https://www.hsph.harvard.edu/nutritionsource/2016/07/05/different-dietary-fat-different-risk-of-mortality/.

209 Eggen, Douglas A., Jack P. Strong, William P. Newman, Gray T. Malcom, and Carlos Restrepo. "Regression of experimental atherosclerotic lesions in rhesus monkeys consuming a high saturated fat diet." Arteriosclerosis: An Official Journal of the American Heart Association, Inc. 7, no. 2 (1987): 125-134.

210 "Heart Disease Facts." Centers for Disease Control and Prevention. https://www.cdc.gov/heartdisease/facts.htm.

211 Mary Ellen Shoup. "Pizza Hut adds 25% more cheese to pan pizzas as part of dairy checkoff program." March 1, 2018. Dairyreporter.com. https://www.dairyreporter.com/Article/2018/03/01/Pizza-Hut-adds-25-more-cheese-to-pan-pizzas-as-part-of-dairy-checkoff-program.

212 Lauren Hirsch. "Kraft Heinz agrees to buy paleo mayo and dressing company Primal Kitchen." November 29, 2018. CNBC.

213 Wilson, Edward O. *Consilience: The unity of knowledge*. Vol. 31. Vintage, 1999.

214 McIlvain, Helen E., Elisabeth L. Backer, Benjamin F. Crabtree, and Naomi Lacy. "Physician attitudes and the use of office-based activities for tobacco control." *FAMILY MEDICINE-KANSAS CITY-* 34, no. 2 (2002): 114-119.

215 Doll, Richard, Richard Peto, Keith Wheatley, Richard Gray, and Isabelle Sutherland. "Mortality in relation to smoking: 40 years' observations on male British doctors." *Bmj* 309, no. 6959 (1994): 901-911.

Made in the USA
Middletown, DE
31 August 2020